IN HIS GRIP

IN HIS GRIP
MEDITATIONS WITH THE GREAT PHYSICIAN
published by Stronghold Press, Dallas, Texas 75238.

© 2011 by Joe and Terri Fornear
ISBN 978-0-98401-131-5

Cover photograph by Rebecca Horn
Book design by rhorngraphics

Stronghold Press
Dallas, Texas 75238
www.mystronghold.org

IN HIS GRIP

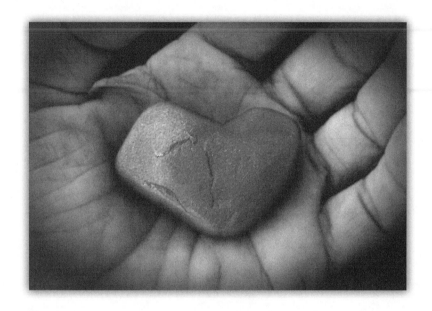

MEDITATIONS
with the
GREAT PHYSICIAN

by joe and terri fornear

STRONGHOLD
PRESS

CONTENTS

♡

INTRODUCTION

♡

Do you not know? Have you not heard? The Everlasting God, the LORD, the Creator of the ends of the earth does not become weary or tired. His understanding is inscrutable. He gives strength to the weary. And to him who lacks might He increases power. Though youths grow weary and tired, and vigorous young men stumble badly, yet those who wait for the LORD will gain new strength; they will mount up with wings like eagles, they will run and not get tired, they will walk and not become weary

(Isaiah 40:28-31).

There is a crucial revelation in the life of every baby eagle. It comes at a most opportune time—during a free-fall to the ground. Utter panic sets in as it tries to prevent its plunge to earth. To slow its fall, it seeks to eject the two "weights" that have been dangling at its sides. Eventually the eaglet discovers their true purpose—the weights are wings which capture air and create lift. Soon the eaglet is soaring to heights it could previously only imagine, if not for that terrifying free-fall to earth.

Yet there is a twist on the flight education of eaglets. The misconception is that they learn to fly by accident after tumbling off the edge of the nest. In fact, it is their own mothers who create these "teachable moments," repeatedly dropping them from high altitudes and catching them before impact with the ground. Eventually the eaglet grasps the lesson—its weights are wings.

My (Joe) battle with Stage IV metastatic melanoma in 2002–2003 appeared to be an "appointment with the ground." The writing was on the wall, ceiling and floor. Once melanoma slips past the lymph nodes, it is a major problem. My case was advanced Stage IV, spreading to 13 different sites including lung, kidney, stomach and a mass on both the head and tail of my pancreas. I had a large patch of cancer in the lymph nodes of my pelvis. The growth spread through my pelvis and eventually fractured one of my ischium (sitting) bones. I lost over 60 pounds and was literally on the edge of death. My doctor told me in May 2003 that I had "days to live," but the Lord intervened in dramatic fashion, and snatched me from certain death. My doctor proclaimed the sudden turnaround to be nothing short of a miracle, and I have been cancer free since August 2003!*

---

*See more on my story in the book, *My Stronghold, A Pastor's Battle with Cancer and Doubt.*

The physical side of our journey was, as they say, only half of the battle. Unseen emotional and spiritual forces pummeled us throughout the initial fight. New waves of fierce storms still raged for seven years after being declared cancer free. We were faced with some serious complications from the cancer treatments which required surgery. Also on several heart-stopping occasions we were told erroneously that the cancer had returned. Again and again we have felt the gravity of cancer's clutches jerking us downward—or was it the Lord teaching us to fly?

From impossible altitudes, at least for us, the Lord repeatedly dropped us to reinforce that crucial revelation—our weaknesses are truly strengths. Yet, over and over He reached down to snatch us up before we crashed on rocks of frustration, self-pity and independence. We have found Him to be our Rock and Stronghold, a refuge and a source of great strength in times of trouble. Even when we had begun to lose our grip, too weak to hang on, He has held onto us.

Stronghold Ministry

So what was the Lord trying to accomplish in our lives through these trials? He is always purposeful, and we believe He had a plan in delivering me (Joe) from a sentence of death. Fulfillment of that plan began in late 2008, when I was led to step aside from an 18-year pastorate to launch Stronghold Ministry, which provides spiritual support to cancer patients, their networks and others in crisis. During our cancer battle, we received medical, physical and even emotional support from professionals and lay advisers. Yet there was little spiritual or Scriptural input from those who truly understand how to climb out of the dark shadows of a battle with cancer.

We believe the Bible has so much to offer, but for cancer patients and caretakers, it is a remarkable treasure. So we are not afraid to proclaim, "Thus says the Lord," as we believe He delights in speaking to us through the messages of comfort we call The Scriptures. Stronghold Ministry is unapologetically Christian, centering on the person, words and work of Jesus Christ. The Bible's timeless encouragements still work today. What better way to lift a struggler than to remind them of their Creator's very thoughts towards them? Dealing with cancer is hard enough without trying to handle it alone in a spiritual desert!

Through our ministry and now this book, we share the lessons we gleaned from our battle. Like many others, when faced with a life-threatening disease, we too sought out our Creator with great urgency. Without finding fault for past drifting, God welcomed this depth of relationship with us, just as He welcomes all who turn to Him. It is so true: it is often in crisis that we grow closest to Him.

We come alongside hurting cancer patients and caretakers to help strengthen and encourage them with the comfort and lessons we have received. We re-assure all that it is He who seeks out the weak to show Himself strong on our behalf. We accept the patients, wherever they are in their journey, whether crippled with fear, dripping with resentment or just simply confused. We give what we have freely received:

> Blessed be the God Father of our Lord Jesus Christ, the Father of mercies and God of all comfort, who comforts us in all our affliction so that we will be able to comfort those who are in any affliction with the comfort with which we ourselves are comforted by God. For just as the sufferings of Christ are ours in abundance, so also our comfort is abundant through Christ (2 Corinthians 1:3-5).

Yet seeking to soar above one's troubles is a lifelong lesson. We are painfully aware that our own training is ongoing, and we are mere beginners. When hardships come, we still obsess over ridding ourselves of the burden. Realizing others share our need for continual reminders, we present this book, *In His Grip, Meditations with The Great Physician*. It is a book of short devotional read-ings that each contain a Scripture, a lesson and a prayer. Most of these devo-tionals were distributed on a weekly basis through our *In His Grip* weekly newsletter and blog. Some readings are new, and some date back to the thick of our cancer battle. We have divided 90 devotionals into topical categories, such as God's, Love and Surrender. These topics are listed in the Contents so readers might find and focus on specific issues. Readers may choose to chew on one reading per day or tackle entire sections in one sitting. Our goal is to simply help the readers become aware of and access the Lord's supernatural resources for their journeys. Our hope is that they too will find Him to be a Stronghold in the midst of their troubles.

So we ask you to join with us in lifting up the first of many prayers in this book.

♡

Lord, we ask You to use this book to bring Your Presence, power and comfort to all who read.

GOD'S LOVE

♡

Love Breaks Through

joe fornear

Who will separate us from the love of Christ? Will tribulation, or distress, or persecution, or famine, or nakedness, or peril, or sword? Just as it is written, "For your sake we are being put to death all day long; we were considered as sheep to be slaughtered." But in all these things we overwhelmingly conquer through Him who loved us. For I am convinced that neither death, nor life, nor angels, nor principalities, nor things present, nor things to come, nor powers, nor height, nor depth, nor any other created thing, will be able to separate us from the love of God, which is in Christ Jesus our Lord.

ROMANS 8:35–39

This passage delivers a powerful message to the person struggling with cancer or any major crisis. This is an absolute guarantee in the Lord's response to His children's cries. His love has an air tight grip on us, and nothing, including cancer, death, or any other crisis can prevent us from experiencing His love in Jesus Christ.

Some may react to this section of Romans 8, "I'm certainly not feeling His love right now." But feelings are poor barometers of facts. We should cling to these facts:

God's love is far, far greater than our troubles. Troubles shrink when compared to God's infinite love. "And I pray that you, being rooted and established in love, may have power, together with all the saints, to grasp how wide and long and high and deep is the love of Christ, and to know this love that surpasses knowledge—that you may be filled to the measure of all the fullness of God" (Ephesians 3:17–19).

We *can* experience His love in the midst of any trouble. Don't be guided by unreliable feelings; tell yourself the truth: "I can do all things through Him who strengthens me" (Philippians 4:13).

We "overwhelmingly conquer" through Christ and His love. We can move beyond surviving, to thriving, even in the harshest circumstances. "Now to Him who is able to do immeasurably more than all we ask or imagine, according to His power that is at work within us, to Him be glory" (Ephesians 3:20–21).

So thank Him—no, *praise* Him for the absolute truth of these facts which apply to you now and always. Your praises are an act of faith, and we want to "walk by faith, not by sight," (2 Corinthians 5:7). We don't have to be burdened by upsetting feelings. As you persevere in praise, waves of His love will break through the noise and gloom of difficulties. So look away from your trials to be comforted by the One whose love envelops and grips your soul. Who will separate us from the love of God? Not even you can!

Lord, train us to continually soak up and enjoy Your love which you lavishly pour out on us.

His Shouts of Deliverance

terri fornear

You are my hiding place; you preserve me from trouble, and surround me with shouts of deliverance.

Psalm 32:7

I was working with one of the kids I tutor and in the middle of the lesson he said, "Ms. Terri, did you know we are made of more nothing than something?" He proceeded to tell me how science has proven that cells have more empty space than space that is filled by matter. More nothing than something? At first I laughed. Then I got excited, realizing that Colossians 1:17 says, "In Him all things hold together," and Ephesians 1:23 says of Jesus, "[He] fills all and is in all." This made me think maybe there is more of Him in me, than me, which opens up all kinds of possibilities!

The invisible is becoming more real. What I see is often overwhelming, and out of my control. Talking to an invisible God who holds everything together is a faith walk into the unseen.

Today as I read Psalm 32:7, I repeat His words aloud to Him, "You are my hiding place; you preserve me from trouble, and surround me with shouts of deliverance." I want to hear His "shouts of deliverance."

How do I do that? I have to quiet my heart to hear. What are these "shouts?" I must really "listen," as some make no sound at all.

- Thorns placed on His head (a reminder that He bears the thorns we deal with every day).
- Nails pounded into His hands and feet (delivering me from punishment for my sin).
- The vinegar He drank (drinking the comfort He gives as I let go of my dreams).
- His tears and bloody sweat in Gethsemane (bearing the anxieties, worries and fears of future trials).
- Dragging His cross (so that we could benefit from His Resurrection life today).
- Then finally His last shout, "IT IS FINISHED."

His Resurrected life, though now still invisible, keeps shouting for me to "see" His deliverance in the midst of the visible. Here are more of His shouts:

- "You are complete in me" (Colossians 2:10).
- "I will never leave you" (John 14:18).
- "You are righteous in Me" (Romans 4:8).
- "You are completely forgiven" (1 John 2:9).
- "Enter My rest" (Hebrews 4:3).
- "There is no condemnation for those who are in Me" (Romans 8:1).
- "Take My peace. It is not like the world's peace" (John 14:19).
- "Abide in My unconditional love" (1 John 2:28).
- "Cast your cares on me, for I care for you" (1 Peter 5:7).
- "I will help you overcome the evil one" (1 John 2:13).
- "Greater is He that is in you than he who is in the world" (1 John 4:4).

Keep Yourself in God's Love
joe fornear

How precious also are Your thoughts to me, O God! How vast is the sum of them!
If I should count them, they would outnumber the sand.

Psalm 139:17

When our fight against cancer wracks our body with pain and rubs our emotions raw, it's not easy to focus on God's love for us. At such times, we may be tempted to wonder if God even loves us at all! If He loves us so much, why doesn't He say the word and remove our pain and heal our jangled emotions?

David must have wondered about God's love too. God had anointed him king over Israel in Saul's place, yet David did not fully consolidate his throne for many years. Saul had made finding and killing David his life's priority. David spent years running from Saul. He was driven away to hide and fight for his life in the territory of his other enemies, the Philistines.

Despite the toxic hate that constantly surrounded him, David mastered a mind-set that kept him experiencing God's love. David's secret was his focus. God did not have to circumstantially "prove" His love, by removing Saul from his life. David learned how to tune into the loving whispers of God deep in his spirit. He did not allow Saul or anyone else to steal his sense of God's love.

I love the way my daughter Amy, at the age of 21, wrote about God's love in this Psalm.

Think about all the sand grains in the world at the bottom of the ocean floor, between your toes, sand volleyball, the beach and the sandy edges of lakes, the sand MOUNTAINS in the deserts, the little glass vases filled with sand in people's bathrooms. That is a lot of sand! God thinks about you MORE than the number of sand grains on earth. His thoughts toward you are precious. See Psalm 139 (verse 17).

God's positive thoughts about you outnumber the sand grains in the world! Focus on that and let it soak in deep into your spirit.

♡

Lord, it is sometimes difficult to bask in your love. Help us to draw deep from Your heart full of love for us!

5

Pie in the Sky Now

joe fornear

Things which eye has not seen and ear has not heard, and which have not entered the heart of man,
all that God has prepared for those who love him. For to us God revealed them through
the Spirit; for the Spirit searches all things, even the depths of God. For who among men knows the
thoughts of a man except the spirit of the man which is in him? Even so the thoughts
of God no one knows except the Spirit of God. Now we have received, not the spirit of the world, but
the Spirit who is from God, so that we may know the things freely given to us by God.

1 Corinthians 2:9-12

Bible quiz time. To what time or era do these verses refer? Though some will surely answer, "Heaven," these verses have actually been fulfilled long ago—on earth!

This quote in 1 Corinthians 2:9 is a quotation of Isaiah 64:4, where Isaiah longs for the day when God will reveal what He has in store for those who love Him. Isaiah penned this in 654 B.C. In 1 Corinthians 2, which was written around A.D. 57, Paul declared this day of revelation had come because the Holy Spirit had already begun revealing "the things freely given to us by God" (1 Corinthians 2:12). Note the past tense. He has already given these things, and they were free! God has given us His Spirit, a Guide to explain His deepest thoughts.

What are these "things" which we already possess? From many related passages about His free gifts and resources which are already ours in Christ, here is a short list:

- His love (Romans 5:5).
- His peace (John 14:27).
- His wisdom (James 1:5).
- His joy (John 16:24).
- His comfort (2 Corinthians 1:3–4).

Some might wonder if we can possibly experience these blessings when we're sick. Yet if one considers the context of each of these promises, they've been freely given to those in the midst of great tribulations!

If you believe in the goodness of God, ask yourself, would He allow us to go through hardship and not be your Stronghold through it? Surely He will provide the necessary resources to handle the pain. When I lean on the Lord in my troubles, I find my experience of His goodness is greatest.

"Pie in the sky" does not have to be "by and by." The "things freely given to us by God" and "all that God has prepared for those who love Him" are for our enjoyment now!

Lord, help us depend on You to discover all things that You have prepared for us today!

Hedged In to the Giver

joe fornear

Have You not made a hedge about him and his house and all that he has, on every side?
You have blessed the work of his hands, and his possessions have increased in the land.

Job 1:10

Shall we accept good from God, and not trouble?

Job 2:10

Until recently, some of you may have not experienced much trouble. Big troubles were for others. Then suddenly and without notice, trouble showed up at your door; but this was inevitable. Someone has rightly said, "We are either in trouble, coming out of trouble or heading into trouble." So how do we handle trouble? Job can teach us well.

Job knew that God was good, and that He often demonstrated it through His gifts. Yet Job knew that God's goodness didn't end when His gifts were withdrawn. Everything Job ever touched turned to gold. He was blessed beyond anyone of his time. Satan referred to this charmed life as a "hedge." Yet he accused Job of being faithful to God only because of the gifts. Satan was granted permission by God to break through the hedge to test the objects of Job's affections.

In one day, Job's flocks, herds, servants and all 10 of his beloved children were suddenly and tragically taken away. Then Job's good health was replaced with a horrific skin disease, leaving him shaken to his very core. Still Job maintained an unqualified love for God. "The Lord gives and the Lord takes away, blessed be the name of the Lord" (Job 1:21). And, "Shall we accept good from God, and not trouble?" (Job 2:10). And, "Though He slay me, yet will I love Him" (Job 13:5).

Job's secret was to love and cling to the Giver, not His gifts. Job was actually hedged into God Himself. He fought through the waves of pain and disappointment to latch onto the abiding blessedness of God. We can do this, too. I know it's hard to see when our eyes of faith are so clouded by tears. But what is impossible for us, is possible for us and God.

Jesus knew the sting of feeling forsaken by God. Yet He was not abandoned to despair, and neither are you. Jesus fought through the pain "because of the joy set before Him" (Hebrews 12:2). There is an amazing blessing for those who focus their affections on God alone. Can you say with Job, "Blessed be the name of the Lord"? His love is always freely available to you. Can you sense His love for you, in spite of the pain?

Lord, even now, please pour out an overwhelming sense of your love into our hearts.
Fill us with the warmth of your goodness and give us hearts of praise for You,
because You are always worthy of our praise and affections.

Biting the Hand that Restores You

joe fornear

*Jesus said, "How often I wanted to gather your children together,
just as a hen gathers her brood under her wings, and you would not have it!"*

Luke 13:34

During our friend's battle with cancer, she and her husband had an experience with their dog which was packed with symbolism. Her husband was trying to call the dog to come inside, but it refused to listen. It ran onto the street directly into the path of an oncoming car. The dog was pretty banged up in the collision, but managed to get up and start walking. When his master tried to reach down and scoop it up to nurse it back to health, it bit down viciously on his hand, and then limped off. The dog continued to ignore its master's calls and ran away to hide.

Amazingly, a couple of days later, they found the dog and it allowed them to give the care it needed. All along, the dog's master had its well-being in mind, but the dog perceived it differently, and chose to go it alone. When you see this self-destructive behavior played out in a dog's life, the folly seems so clear. But doesn't this mirror us when we try to handle life apart from God? We get independent, think we know better, drift away and then reject His restoring help.

Just like Adam and Eve in the Garden of Eden, we can be deceived to believe that God is not totally good. The temptation is to believe that He is withholding life's finest blessings. And then when we encounter self-imposed pain, we bite the hand that is reaching to restore us. Yet there is no good reason to run away from the God who loves us. He always has our best in mind. Jesus is very clear in this verse in Luke 13. He wants to protect and nurture us, but we must allow Him.

Today, remember this when you are tempted to drift away: God is really good, all of the time. He has your very best in mind!

*Lord, forgive us for our tendency to drift away,
and remind us that Your loving hands guide us into safety and restoration.*

Can You Hear Him Now?

joe fornear

For while we were still helpless, at the right time Christ died for the ungodly.
For one will hardly die for a righteous man; though perhaps for the good man someone
would dare even to die. But God demonstrates His own love toward us,
in that while we were yet sinners, Christ died for us.

Romans 5:7-9

During times of crisis, a burning question captivates many minds. "Lord, if You really love me, why don't You remove my pain *now*?" Some ask the question innocently and honestly, willing to "listen" to God's response. Some conclude that He is just flat unfair. Some are so confused that they basically suppress the question.

God's ways will not be fully grasped until eternity. In the meantime, there have been countless attempts to resolve this issue. Still, God has left us with one loud, clear statement regarding the scope of His love.

You see, anyone can claim to love, but God has *demonstrated* His love for us in one grand gesture. During my great crisis of Stage IV melanoma, this great act of love was an anchor for me in the midst of my confusion.

For while we were still helpless, at the right time Christ died for the ungodly. For one will hardly die for a righteous man; though perhaps for the good man someone would dare even to die. But God demonstrates His own love toward us, in that while we were yet sinners, Christ died for us (Romans 5:7–9).

Did you catch when Jesus died for us—while we were yet sinners? He made the ultimate sacrifice to prove His unconditional love for us, even though we had proven to be His enemies

If we hold on to this eternal truth, we will not be shaken by current events. As we rest in His arms of love, His hope and peace will prevail. Though we may not *feel* it now, He has proven His love for us. He loves us more than we can even comprehend!

The next time you wonder about His love, remind yourself of the ultimate expression of His love—His intense suffering and dying for the forgiveness for your sin. Yes, He really, really loves you.

Lord, thank You for demonstrating your incredible love to us
by giving Your very best, Your only Son, Jesus Christ.

All-Wise, All-Powerful and Amazingly Tender

joe fornear

And He was saying, "Abba! Father! All things are possible for You;
remove this cup from Me; yet not what I will, but what You will."

Mark 14:36

What a prayer! Jesus knew a few things about our Father, didn't He? The following are some observations about Jesus' understanding of His Father's heart toward Him—and us:

The Father was tender. Jesus called the Father, *"Abba,"* which is like calling Him "Daddy" or "Papa." The Father enjoys intimacy with us. Do you want to have that type of closeness with Him? Do you let Him get that close to you? Open up to Him.

The Father was all powerful. *"All things are possible for You."* During my cancer journey, I had seen enough of Stage IV metastatic melanoma to know it was bigger than me and modern medicine as well. Still, a thought kept bolstering my sense of well-being: cancer is absolutely no match for God Almighty. He can do anything as nothing is too hard for Him. He could snap His finger and make it all go away in a split second. For me, that stripped ALL of cancer's power. He always has the last word.

The Father's will is best. *"Yet not what I will, but what You will."* Jesus was content to yield to His Father's final decision. Still He prayed three times for *"the cup to pass."* He was hoping to avoid crucifixion and also "becoming sin for us" (2 Corinthians 5:21). Jesus asked for some other way to accomplish man's redemption.

Yet Jesus knew if the Father asked Him to go through with the crucifixion that the Father would be there for Him. Even though He felt forsaken for a time, the joy of their relationship would soon be restored. So we can rest in His power, decisions and heart toward us, while not fearing ANY outcome. He is good.

Lord, open our eyes to Your awesome power and tender heart.

COPING
with
HARDSHIP

♡

How to Handle "One of Those Days"

joe fornear

The LORD is good, a stronghold in the day of trouble.
And He knows those who take refuge in Him.

Nahum 1:7

At some point in our lives, we will all endure a "day of trouble." Wouldn't it be nice if troubles lasted just one day or 24 hours? In the Hebrew language, "day" can mean some indefinite period of time, which some have called a "season." Perhaps you find yourself in a season of "one of those days," even a long fight against cancer. There is plenty of hope for you, however, because those who turn to the Lord find great relief. Nahum 1:7 provides three key lessons on how to handle the day of trouble.

Trust the goodness of the Lord during our trials. Nahum first focuses on the goodness of God, not the trial. "The Lord is good." He is always good, and we can access His goodness as He pours out comfort, assurance and peace. Perhaps our greatest error is to equate His goodness with His removal of our trials. We mistakenly reason, "God, if You're good, You will remove this trouble for me—now." Trust Him; He has other ways to arrive at our ultimate good.

Lean on Him during trials. The term "stronghold" is a military term describing a fortified city that was well-defended and hard to breach. When used of God, it is a reference to His mighty protection and strength. He guards our hearts from spiritual attacks such as fear, self-pity, condemnation and doubts. He provides a "refuge" or shelter from any storm.

He certainly held me up during my fierce battle with Stage IV metastatic melanoma. In May 2003, after being given days to live, I had become so weakened by surgeries, treatments, and being human, that I found myself losing my grip. As I cried out to Him, He reminded me that though I was out of control, He wasn't. Though I was worried, He wasn't. He had a firm grip on me, and I found Him to be a powerful Stronghold. This is why we named our ministry to cancer patients, Stronghold Ministry, in honor of His promise to carry us through days of trouble.

Answer the Lord's invitation to an ever-deepening relationship with Him. Nahum uses an intriguing phrase here, that the Lord "knows those who take refuge in Him." This reminds me of Psalm 139 where God tells us He knows everything about us. His thoughts are not only countless, but precious toward us. As we turn to Him, He reveals Himself to be an incredible companion throughout our journeys.

Think for a moment of a human hero of yours. It is one thing to know all about your hero, but it is quite another when he knows everything about you! Nothing could be better than to be personally "known" by God Himself! He knows *you*.

So when you're confused and frustrated in your day of trouble, turn to Him, not away from Him. You're not alone. He is good, and He is your Stronghold in the day of trouble.

Lord, thank You for being so good to us, all of the time!

Always Good News

joe fornear

Do not be afraid of sudden fear.
Proverbs 3:25

How does one stay positive when you're flooded with bad news? Is your doctor continually giving reports of serious health problems? Do you have "scanxiety" about an upcoming test?

I can't say I've mastered a positive mind-set. I've been known to throw a tantrum simply because of a traffic jam. Still, in my life and in the lives of many others, I have seen the power of God lift the human spirit, even in the bleakest circumstances.

You see, God is not just a nice idea, HE IS A LIVING GOD! He delights in showing up when we are at the bottom. He allows humbling trials and chronic weaknesses to show us how strong He can be on our behalf.

Consider and take Him up on these offers:

Peace. He promises a "peace that surpasses all understanding" in Philippians 4:7. What does this mean? It's the type of peace where people marvel at how in the world someone can remain so calm. This peace is "not of this world," as Jesus says in John 14:27, it is supernaturally provided and based on God's control over the universe and not the smoothness of our circumstances.

Love. In Ephesians 3:9, He promises we can experience a "love which surpasses knowledge that you may be filled up to all the fullness of God." This means the love of God will go above and beyond our minds to our hearts and feelings. We can actually be filled with warm, uplifting love, not just intellectually aware of the fact He loves us.

Joy. And joy, oh that elusive joy. Everyone wants it. God provides it. For free. Jesus said in John 15:11, "These things I have spoken to you so that My joy may be in you, and that your joy may be made full." This joy is not only from God, it is *His* joy. I don't think God gets down in the dumps. I'll gladly take His joy over anyone else's.

So no matter what news comes your way, look for His supernaturally supplied resources to cope.

Lord, thank You for providing resources so powerful that they overshadow my circumstances.

Rest Stop

joe fornear

Come to Me, all who are weary and heavy-laden, and I will give you rest.
Take My yoke upon you and learn from Me, for I am gentle and humble in heart, and you
will find rest for your souls. For My yoke is easy and My burden is light.

Matthew 11:28

Everyone gets weary due to life's day-to-day demands. So it's not surprising we're overwhelmed when we find ourselves in a life-threatening crisis. Where do we turn? Some say, "When you're at the end of your rope, tie a knot and hang on." Yet that assumes one has the strength to hold on while tying a knot! In contrast, Jesus says, "You can let go of the rope, I have a firm hold on you. Why are you trying to climb this rope alone anyway?" He offers serious relief in Matthew 11:28, and gives three directives which lead to genuine rest for the hurting soul:

Come to Me. Sometimes we allow pain and exhaustion to turn us away from the Lord. Sometimes our drift is fueled by anger and evident, "I don't remember signing up for this." Or we may nurse a low-grade anger toward God. We're afraid to question or vent at God, so we grow increasingly indifferent toward Him. Yet it's never too late to turn back to Him. He always gladly welcomes us back. So throw the weight of your burdens, fears and concerns on Him. Go to Him.

Take My yoke upon you. A yoke is a leather and wood harness fastened to oxen to pull a plow. When Jesus tells us to take His yoke upon us, He's referring to a double yoke. Older, stronger oxen were partnered with clumsy, young ox, and of course the older ox did the heavy lifting. Jesus wants to team up with each of us to tackle our day's burdens. Compared to our frantic and frustrated efforts, He promises to make our lives "easy" and the pulling "light." We weren't designed to pull solo, especially in a crisis, so let Him lighten your load.

Be meek and humble. Sometimes independence is our greatest enemy. Perhaps we even wish to take credit for making it through alone. This is probably why He emphasizes meekness and humility in this passage: "I am meek and humble of heart." Meekness is toward man; not seeking to be someone great or superior. Humility is toward God; not wanting to control our own lives, but yielding over to Him who knows much more.

Many of our burdens are self-imposed. The heaviest weights we carry are not health or financial concerns, but ego and pride. I'm glad Jesus meets us when we're at the end of our ropes. Simply rest in Him.

Lord, You are so gracious to desire to carry our load alongside of us.
Help us learn how to share the load with You.

Difficulty Factors
joe fornear

God does not ignore the suffering of the afflicted.
He does not hide his face but listens to the cry for help.

Psalm 22:24

In Olympic diving competition, dives are rated according to "difficulty factor." There is a built-in acknowledgment that some dives are more complicated than others. In so many cancer battles I've observed, with all of the physical, emotional and financial challenges, the difficulty factor is sky high. Yet the Lord can help us survive, and even thrive, in the midst of fighting cancer.

Some thoughts on handling the difficulty factors:

Realize the Lord notices *your* **difficulties.** "God does not ignore the suffering of the afflicted. He does not hide his face but listens to the cry for help" (Psalm 22:24). This promise helped when my cancer battle was at its fiercest. He did not immediately stop my suffering, but He let me know He was there—and He cared. He knows our journeys are hard. Fortunately, as the verse implies, He doesn't just watch from the sidelines.

Superhuman challenges require supernatural resources. You probably noticed how quickly your human endurance and strength wear down. Fortunately, we can ask the Lord for His strength. He knows we're in over our heads, and waits for us to ask. He offers supernatural help and we should take it!

He has given us His peace to weather the storm. "My peace I give to you; not as the world gives do I give to you. Do not let your heart be troubled, nor let it be fearful" (John 14:27). His peace is not tied to circumstances. His peace surpasses understanding (Philippians 4:7). Do you think Jesus Christ is ever worried or fearful?

Know your limitations. Some of us are driven and over-responsible, but when we are in a crisis, we must learn to say no. When we're battling, or helping someone battle cancer, we will probably have to focus more time and energy than we would like on getting well or helping someone get well. Some regular tasks, and even important ones will not get done, and that is just fine. We must pace ourselves as we are not machines!

Lose the attitudes and grudges. Nothing drains us faster than negativity. A bad attitude draws the vitality right out of our environment. When we focus on complaining, we strengthen self-pity, and our problems become bigger than they really are. We may even grant them a position higher than God! When we hold grudges, we hold our well-being hostage to those who hurt us. Yet God is greater than any hurt or pain. So focus on forgiving everyone (yes, everyone), and you will experience more of the Lord's gracious freedom in you.

Ask for human help. People always tell cancer patients, "Let me know if there is anything I can do." So go ahead and give folks specific ways to help you! If no one is offering, call on someone and ask for help. One of our Stronghold Ministry patients has shared some good advice, "Never be too proud to ask for help when the burden is too heavy to bear alone, for courage often requires humility."

Lord, thank You for coming alongside us and walking us through the great difficulty of battling cancer.

Do You Hear What I Hear?

joe fornear

*But if any of you lacks wisdom, let him ask of God, who gives to all generously
and without reproach, and it will be given to him. But he must ask in faith without any doubting,
for the one who doubts is like the surf of the sea, driven and tossed by the wind.
For that man ought not to expect that he will receive anything from the Lord,
being a double-minded man, unstable in all his ways.*

James 1:5-8

When you're fighting cancer, advice abounds. Everywhere you turn, someone is telling you about a supplement, book or treatment that will help you beat cancer. This is not always a bad thing, as the Lord often uses the advice of others to steer us. For so many, the stakes are really high, and the options and opinions are numerous. The sense of responsibility can be unnerving. During my battle, I often struggled with what to do next. Fortunately, the Lord promises to weigh in.

In God's birth announcement of His Son in Isaiah 9:6, He refers to Jesus as the "Wonderful Counselor." This attribute of Jesus provides lasting benefits for all who follow Him. He is the gift-who-keeps-on-giving. Could you use some Divine counseling to navigate today's decisions?

God delighted to share His wisdom with those in crisis in the Old and New Testament. His promise to supply specific guidance is still good today. He will lead us through anything we face, from treatment options to how to cope with the spiritual and emotional upheaval of our battle.

So how does He guide today? I wouldn't expect an audible voice, but do expect that when you ask, one way or another, He will provide the wisdom you need. He promises.

He may "speak" through a Bible verse which seems to "jump off the page." Keep in mind that He never leads us contrary to His objective Word, the Bible, so it is important to grow in using it for guidance.

He also speaks through wise, godly people. He speaks through doctors, nurses and fellow warriors. Proverbs 15:22 tells us, "Without consultation, plans are frustrated, but with many counselors they succeed." So go ahead and gather much experienced advice.

You may possibly hear from Him through a stranger who is an angel in human disguise. I have had a few experiences that I supposed were angelic encounters. Hebrews 13:2 reminds us, "Do not neglect to show hospitality to strangers, for by this some have entertained angels without knowing it."

James 1:5–8 tells us to ask in faith, believing that He not only *can* lead us, but that He *will* lead us. So here is how I make big decisions. I gather all of the input from many sources. I take them to the Lord and ask Him to guide me to the best option. Then I trust He is guiding me when I decide what seems best. Some might say this is just common sense. I say it is *sanctified* common sense in that the living God is intentionally drawn into the process and He loves to be asked for His opinion.

> Trust in the LORD with all your heart and do not lean on your own under-standing. In all your ways acknowledge Him, and He will make your paths straight. Do not be wise in your own eyes; Fear the LORD and turn away from evil. It will be healing to your body and refreshment to your bones (Proverbs 3:5–8).

The Bible describes a close personal relationship with a God who cares. We will grow in learning how to "hear" Him as we habitually tune in each day. He will either change our circumstances or provide us with a path to peacefully manage those circumstances. Either way, He's on our side, and He delights to lead us. So listen up! Do you hear what I hear?

Lord, thank You that You delight to help lead us in our greatest decisions.

The Survivor's New Normal

joe fornear

"For I know the plans that I have for you," declares the LORD, "plans for welfare and not for calamity to give you a future and a hope."

Jeremiah 29:11

This may be surprising, but it is common for cancer survivors to struggle with depression *after* being declared cancer free. Now you might wonder, "They had their prayers answered, so what could possibly be the problem?" Many people expect survivors to be all chirpy and happy, but they may not play the part.

From 1980 to 2010, the number of cancer survivors in the United States has tripled and is growing by two percent each year. From those trends, there were almost 15 million cancer survivors, representing five percent of the United States population. Yet oncologists and psychologists are only now becoming aware how common it is for survivors to fight with mild to moderate depression.

Drawing from my own experience and also other warriors we've encountered in our ministry, I'd like to offer several reasons genuine happiness can elude the survivor. Then I'd like to suggest some biblical advice on how to handle these post-war blues.

Fear. Immediately after being declared cancer free, the thought that the cancer could recur is never far from consciousness. Fear lies in wait and rears up at the first sign of a pain or lump.

Adrenaline letdown. For many, there is a sort of post-traumatic stress syndrome (PTSD) after a cancer battle. Returning to "civilian life" is not as easy as one might think. Many patients literally fought for their life. They were all jacked up on adrenaline and constantly on guard. After the battle, it is truly difficult to relax. Emotional recovery takes time as well.

Literal battle scars. Surgeries, chemo and radiation take their toll and leave their marks. The potential list of scars is lengthy: neuropathy from chemo (painful tingling of nerves in fingers, toes and feet), burns from radiation, loss of limb function, weight loss or gain and lasting side effects from many medications. Withdrawal from mood-altering pain management drugs can be another factor in being down. For personal or privacy reasons, some scars may never be shared by survivors, such as issues pertaining to sexual function or body image issues.

Figurative battle scars. Battle fatigue is often rampant among survivors. Chemo and other drugs depress the immune and nervous systems, so it is no wonder they depress the emotions as well. Grieving lost time and opportunities with loved ones is very common. Flashback memories can haunt the survivor, especially at first. Often sadness due to continued or new tensions in relationships impacts the survivor as well. Normalizing relationships after cancer is not easy and takes time.

Purposelessness. The survivor often is paralyzed by big picture questions, "What does this all mean? How should I live now?" Life after cancer can prove so mundane, empty, boring and vacant. Priorities now must be realigned back to "normal," and survivors are often uncertain how to define their "new normal."

Support system changes. Supporters understandably move on, leaving the survivor to process the aftermath of cancer on their own. I really wanted and needed to talk, but I soon realized that not everyone had the time or desire to listen to me process my trauma. Expectations from work, spouse and life returned like a flood, making it clear to me that the kid gloves were off. The message was to pull it together and look to contribute fully again.

So what advice does the Bible give to handle these factors?

Pray and Trust. The Bible says to cast our anxiety on the Lord (1 Peter 5:17). Jesus said we can't add even one day to our lives, so we should trust Him completely with our longevity.

Number your days. Moses said, "Teach us to number our days, that we may present to You a heart of wisdom" (Psalm 90:12). Moses suggests we make each day count for God. Following the Lord on a daily, even a moment-by-moment basis, is wise living advice for all. The martyred missionary, Jim Elliot, once said, "He is no fool who gives what he cannot keep, to gain what he can never lose."

Talk or write it out. Find a support group or some other survivors and talk things over. One of the most healing steps for me was to write a book. I wasn't sure anyone would ever read it, but I felt I had to write it to process my thoughts. Some people journal or write prayers to the Lord. These activities can help to make sense of the entire experience. Reading others' stories helps me. If you are a survivor, contact us (Appendix III) and I will send you my book, *My Stronghold, A Pastor's Battle with Cancer and Doubts*, perhaps it will help you.

Practice the Presence of God. There is no one who can heal our hurts and memories like the Lord. He can "restore the years the locusts have eaten" (Joel 2:25). In other words, He can make up for our losses and lost time. I think the best way He does this is by making each moment special with Him and others.

The Lord, who was my Stronghold in the midst of the storm, can continually hold you up even after the storm blows over.

Lord, we're so grateful that You heal and restore us to new levels of normal with You.

Long May You Run

joe fornear

Then the hand of the LORD was on Elijah, and he girded up his loins and outran Ahab to Jezreel.
1 Kings 18:46

Many trials are marathons, not sprints. Fighting cancer can be lengthy and extremely draining. During the marathon journeys of Elijah the prophet, he was all over the geographical and emotional map (1 Kings 17–19). While fleeing from Queen Jezebel who was full of vengeance toward him, he visited Mt. Carmel, Jezreel, Beersheba, Mt. Sinai (Mt. Horeb) and finally some place in the middle of the desert.

Emotionally, Elijah "visited" supreme confidence and sheer panic; exhilaration and utter exhaustion; outlandish boldness and cowardly surrender. No wonder James said in his epistle that "Elijah was a man with a nature just like ours" (James 5:17). The Greek word James used here is a compound word from "like" and "feelings." In other words, Elijah rode the same emotional roller coaster that we ride today.

Still the Lord accompanied Elijah everywhere he went, to every geographical and emotional peak and valley. On one occasion, Elijah received supernatural strength from the Lord for a long journey (1 Kings 18:46). God's strengthening hand was so heavy upon him that he was able to outrun Ahab's chariot over a distance of 25 miles—and this during a torrential rainstorm! Later, after Elijah had exhausted his strength running from Jezebel, the Lord gave him food that strengthened him for 40 days and 40 nights in the wilderness!

So what is the point for us? James is simply encouraging us that God grants extraordinary answers to prayer. He wants to work great endurance and miraculous energy into our lives. So during the long grind of an up-and-down battle with cancer, we can continually ask for that supernatural infusion of His mighty strength. The Lord will meet us at every place we find ourselves, just as He did with Elijah.

♡

Lord, teach us not to run away and exhaust ourselves when we are scared,
but to run toward Your comforting arms.

SURRENDER

♡

Raise the White Flag or Raise the Roof

joe fornear

The crowd rose up together against them, and the chief magistrates tore their robes off them and proceeded to order them to be beaten with rods. When they had struck them with many blows, they threw them into prison, commanding the jailer to guard them securely; and he, having received such a command, threw them into the inner prison and fastened their feet in the stocks. But about midnight Paul and Silas were praying and singing hymns of praise to God, and the prisoners were listening to them.

Acts 16:22-25

When you think of "surrender," what comes to mind? Giving up? Losing? Waving the white flag? Paul and Silas provided an astounding example of *biblical* surrender in Acts 16. God desires surrender from His children. The type of surrender He seeks includes a joyful willingness to undergo hardship.

Paul and Silas had freed a slave girl from a spirit which enabled her to predict the future (Acts 16). This should have made everyone happy, but her masters were furious to lose their source of great profit. So they stirred up public opinion against Paul and Silas, who were beaten "many blows" with rods. They were imprisoned in a city jail and their feet placed in stocks.

As they sat in the dirt of a darkened dungeon, they surely felt the sting and throbbing of many welts. Instead of complaining or plotting their escape, we are told they began "praying and singing hymns of praise to God, and the other prisoners were listening to them." What an amazing response to vicious mistreatment and injustice! They surely were empowered by the power of the Holy Spirit to enable them to display such a superhuman attitude.

Crises would be so much more tolerable if we praised our way through them. Responding joyfully really is a choice. We tend to think our circumstances dictate our moods. Bad events "make" us unhappy, but with Christ we can rise above circumstances and human emotions.

Perhaps this is part of what Jesus meant by giving us a peace that is not of this world. "Peace I leave with you; My peace I give to you; not as the world gives do I give to you. Do not let your heart be troubled, nor let it be fearful (John 14:27). Note that Jesus tells us "do not let" your heart be troubled or fearful. Can we "make" our emotions obey? Yes! We can *choose* to be peaceful. With His grace and help, we can surrender control of our emotions to the Lord!

What happens next to Paul and Silas?

> And suddenly there came a great earthquake, so that the foundations of the prison house were shaken; and immediately all the doors were opened and everyone's chains were unfastened. When the jailer awoke and saw the prison doors opened, he drew his sword and was about to kill himself, supposing that the prisoners had escaped. But Paul cried out with a loud voice, saying, "Do not harm yourself, for we are all here!" And the jailer called for lights and rushed in, and trembling with fear he fell down before Paul and Silas, and after he brought them out, he said, "Sirs, what must I do to be saved?"
>
> They said, "Believe in the Lord Jesus, and you will be saved, you and your household" (Acts 16:26–31).

The level of Paul and Silas' surrender goes even deeper. A great earthquake shook the prison's foundations, all the doors were opened and all of the prisoner's chains were unfastened. Most followers of Christ would probably surmise that God wanted them to quickly escape. Certainly the jailer expected everyone to run. In those days, prison guards were immediately killed if anyone escaped on their watch. So knowing his eventual fate, the guard drew his sword to end his own life sooner than later. But Paul and Silas quickly convinced him to not harm himself, as their praises and prayers had so mellowed the other prisoners that not even one escaped!

The jailer was overwhelmed by such grace extended his way. He too had become spiritually awakened by Paul and Silas' praise session, and he thirsted for the relationship with God which they enjoyed. "What must I do to be saved?" (Acts 16:30). Biblical surrender not only benefits us, but it often creates hunger in others.

We live in a cultural environment that idolizes comfort. Millions of inventors and engineers spend their entire lives dreaming up ways to make our lives easier. Yet no matter how hard we try, we will never design trouble out of our existence. Jesus said, "These things I have spoken to you, so that in Me you may have peace. In the world you have tribulation, but take courage; I have overcome the world" (John 16:33). The Lord allows tribulations but provides for the overcoming of them *in* Him. Though it's certainly appropriate to pursue human relief, we have great impact on others if we place God's glory above all things, even our own comfort and plans.

Have you been called to suffer physically? You have the daily choice to embrace the suffering or fuss and complain. God stands ready to recruit true followers whose comfort takes a back seat to glorifying Him. During my cancer battle, I admit there were days when I certainly wasn't surrendered. Though I wasn't complaining outwardly, there were days I was just numb to Him and indifferent. Yet the Lord constantly reminded me that He had a plan. I was encouraged that my suffering was never in vain. I could surrender to His higher purposes for my pain.

One doesn't have to have a medical condition to practice surrender. Surrender is required to live with and love that imperfect person in your home. Perhaps you need surrender to be kind to an obnoxious co-worker? Ironically, without surrender victorious living escapes us.

Lord, we want to have greater impact on those around us, so in the midst of our pain, help us surrender to You in Your plans.

Stop Being Good: When the Good Becomes the Enemy of the Best

joe fornear

Now as they were traveling along, He entered a village; and a woman named Martha welcomed Him into her home. She had a sister called Mary, who was seated at the Lord's feet, listening to His word. But Martha was distracted with all her preparations; and she came up to Him and said, "Lord, do You not care that my sister has left me to do all the serving alone? Then tell her to help me." But the Lord answered and said to her, "Martha, Martha, you are worried and bothered about so many things; but only one thing is necessary, for Mary has chosen the good part, which shall not be taken away from her."

Luke 10:38-42

Guess who's coming to visit? Do you think you might panic a little if your hero was coming to your home? When I was a boy, my father's aunt would occasionally visit from another state. She was very kind to us and we "rolled out the red carpet" for her. Once when she arrived, she gushed over how clean and beautiful the house looked. I was about six years old at the time, and told her the truth, "That's because we have been cleaning it for two whole days!" Imagine the preparations you would have if your guest was the Messiah!

Most of us can relate to Martha. She wanted to convey the value she had for her special guest. She wanted everything to be just right. Surely He would notice. So why was He so unimpressed? He ignored her, and lavished attention on that "lazy" Mary, who was just sitting at His feet—doing nothing. So Martha appealed to Jesus to correct Mary, and Jesus rebuked her instead.

What a study in contrasts! Martha demanded Jesus listen to her; Mary listened intently to Jesus. Martha was working out her agenda, while Mary awaited orders. Martha was a list person; Mary was a led person. Martha sulked over her plight; Mary savored His kindness.

With whom do you identify? Are you driven to fulfill some set of internal or external expectations? Are you wearing yourself out being a "good" mother, a "good" caretaker, or a "good" patient? Internal expectations, imposed upon ourselves, are often more demanding than external expectations because "the judge" is *always* present.

In the course of our lives, there are "good" things that must be done, but not to the exclusion of the "best" thing. So go ahead and do good; but to experience life's best, carve out quality and daily time to sit with Jesus. He is alive, and He longs to be with you! He will free you from unnecessary burdens which are wearing you out. His Words will give you peace and comfort. Just sit and listen.

Lord, help us see the freedom and superiority of choosing time with You over our to-do lists.

Get Tough and Surrender

joe fornear

*The LORD your God who goes before you will Himself fight on your behalf,
just as He did for you in Egypt before your eyes.*

Deuteronomy 1:30

There are two types of surrender. One is passive and hopeless; the other is active and hopeful. We must never forget that the Lord is engaged and eager to step in on our behalf. When facing a major trial, like cancer, there is no greater step we can take than surrender. Not surrender to the disease, but yielding to our Creator and His direction. Think for a moment: how could we possibly navigate this battle better than Him? He is the ultimate general and a powerful commander, and His soldiers struggle when they set off on their own.

While staring down Goliath, David knew winning the match was greater than his abilities, but that God's abilities were greater still. "All those gathered here will know that it is not by sword or spear that the LORD saves; for the battle is the LORD's, and He will give all of you into our hands" (1 Samuel 17:47). David knew it didn't matter how tough he was. The Lord would gain the victory.

Yet surrender is not passive; it is not even active—it is proactive. Our highest priority is to stay in close contact with Him, yielding, listening and responding. The Lord will then orchestrate our fight and show us our role step-by-step. Don't worry about making a perfect connection with Him, He always finds a way to lead us. So relax in Him and lean on Him. He is fighting for you and with you.

During my encounter with Stage IV metastatic melanoma, especially at the beginning of the battle, I resisted surrendering to the Lord. I didn't want to have cancer, and stubbornly tried to cling to my usual routines. I was determined to show myself and others that I was tough, as if I could will away the effects of the disease and treatments. My strategy backfired and my health declined even faster. My surrender took the form of listening to the doctors and to my wife.

Once I surrendered, I was much more peaceful, and so were those who were trying to help me!

Get tough in your battles and surrender to the Lord. It's the best strategy.

Lord, impress upon us how much tougher we become when we surrender to let You fight our battles.

Center Point

joe fornear

And He went a little beyond them, and fell on His face and prayed, saying,
"My Father, if it is possible, let this cup pass from Me; yet not as I will, but as You will."

Matthew 26:39

Do you think God's will should be pleasant? Do you think His will should be easy to carry out?

During my battle with cancer, I remember conversations with a valet attendant at the chemo center. The first day he helped me out of the car, he said, "Wow, this is really cramping your style." I assumed he was thinking I was young and full of plans, and this was the last place I wanted to be. He was, of course, correct. At my arrival for another round of chemo, he told me, "Now go up there and tell those doctors and nurses that you have more important things to do." I knew he empathized with me, but he continually raised the question that I could not shake. Why is this happening?

I had given my life to Christ 22 years before I was diagnosed. I had always told the Lord, "I completely surrender my life to You. I trust you, so do what You want with me." My resolve would be severely tested. As my treatments became more intense, the daily activities I loved were set aside. I missed several big events with my teenage kids. My outlets came to a screeching halt; no basketball, fishing or barbecues out on the deck. I could not even preach on Sunday mornings, which was not only my occupation, but my passion.

This was all very difficult for me to handle. I felt trapped and unfulfilled. More than once I told the Lord, "I want my life back." Yet He did not comply. I came to realize I was fixated on my purposes and pursuits and not on His plans for me. By bucking my circumstances, I was resisting God Himself.

Then it dawned on me that my cancer journey was right in the center of His will. This was not some bothersome detour or distraction; this was the primary path He had ordained for me to walk. My sense of relief soared.

Ironically, surrendering to His will gave me more peace and energy than my pastimes ever produced.

God's will for you may be crowded with troubles right now. Let Jesus help you center yourself in surrender to His will. Keep in mind, He knows how to surrender. He was asked by his Father to take a path He would not have chosen. Jesus learned to overcome His own reluctance to submit to the Father's will! What better place can we be than in the center of God's will?

Lord, please give us the wisdom and the strength to surrender to Your perfect will.

Who's Counting?

joe fornear

*Then his wife said to him, "Do you still hold fast your integrity? Curse God and die!"
But he said to her, "You speak as one of the foolish women speaks. Shall we indeed accept good
from God and not accept adversity?"*

Job 2:9-10

(This was written by Joe within weeks of being diagnosed with Stage IV metastatic melanoma.)

A few weeks ago I was talking to my seven-year-old niece. She told me she had eight blessings that day. I said, "Oh yeah, name them," and she ticked off eight good things that happened that day. I was impressed and reminded that counting blessings is a powerful mood-altering exercise. Consider taking a moment now to list eight blessings that you have had today. Now doesn't that brighten you up? We always have much to celebrate.

But sometimes it seems easier to count and recount the trials that pile up on us. Job experienced such overwhelming tragedy that his wife basically advised him, "Job, give it up! Curse God, and maybe He will punish you by taking your life. That is one way to end your misery." One can certainly empathize with her grief. She too had experienced the death of all 10 of their children, and the destruction of their fortune—all on the same day. Soon after, Job contracted a horrible skin disease that caused excruciating pain. This was not exactly material for the annual Christmas letter.

I think Job's story is highlighted in the Bible to show us a human who maintained a good attitude after facing some of the worst Satan could dish out (with God's permission). Satan is toothless compared to the power of self-pity. We must realize that self-pity is one of our most formidable foes. It takes us down a path of self-absorption, isolation and leads to rationalization of sinful reactions. Giving in to self-pity is like voluntarily checking yourself into the city jail.

Job is an example of how to handle the temptation of self-pity. He said, "Shall we indeed accept good from God and not accept adversity." Job basically had the following mind-set: "I am the clay, He is the potter. I will submit myself to Him. He has been so good to me. If He decides that I should go through hardship, how can I grumble at Him? God is good, and He is good all of the time."

My family and I are facing adversity with my recent diagnosis of the dreaded "c-word"—cancer. Doctors have not yet determined what kind of cancer it is, but He who allows us to suffer has a higher purpose—just as He did with Job. In the end, Job counted even more blessings after God prospered him again. So let's "count it all joy when trials and tribulations come our way" (James 1:3–4), for God is working His higher purposes so that He can bring more blessings into our lives. We can count on it!

Lord, in the midst of our adversity, help us count the multitude of ways You have blessed us.

MASTERING EMOTIONS

♡

Seeing Through the Tears

joe fornear

When she had said this, she turned around and saw Jesus standing there,
and did not know that it was Jesus. Jesus said to her, "Woman, why are you weeping?
Whom are you seeking?" Supposing Him to be the gardener, she said to Him, "Sir, if you have carried
Him away, tell me where you have laid Him, and I will take Him away." Jesus said to her,
"Mary!" She turned and said to Him in Hebrew, "Rabboni!" (which means, Teacher).

John 20:14-16

This passage describes a historic moment—the first human encounter with the risen Lord Jesus Christ. By the end of Mary's meeting with Jesus, we are uplifted by the happy reunion. But the scene holds a key lesson for us, so that we might avoid Mary's "mistake." She was so gripped by sadness that she didn't realize she was talking with the very One she sought. This causes me to chuckle at her, but I laugh at myself as well. How often my reactions to minor hardship are just like Mary's response!

Emotions are good and beautiful. They add color and dimension to life. Though emotions can be negatively leveraged by sin, they are patterned after God's attributes. We are, after all, created in His image or after His own personal specifications. Yet if emotions are not steered by His truth, they betray our judgment and fog our view of reality.

It is common for people who love God to feel detached and alone. Elijah had boldly stepped out in faith during an intense confrontation with the false prophets of the evil Queen Jezebel (1 Kings 18 & 19). He had won a decisive battle with the queen, and it was obvious to all that the Lord was on his side. Still, a flaming arrow of doubt somehow pierced him to the core. What if the Lord could not or would not continue to protect him from the vengeance of the queen? He followed his shaky feelings and not his faith, and fled deep into the wilderness, not even stopping to rest for an entire day. He was so depressed he asked the Lord to take his life. In his isolation, he imagined he was the only person of his time who was genuinely serving the Lord. But the Lord told him his estimate was way off. Despite the darkness of the times, there were actually 7,000 people who had remained true to God. Elijah's emotions proved to be a faulty measure of reality.

So just like Mary, Elijah's unchecked emotions skewed his perception of God. He suffered needless fears and distress. Thank God that He has us in His grip and doesn't abandon us to our misconceptions. Just as Jesus revealed Himself through Mary's tears, God broke through Elijah's fears. He fed Elijah; forced him to rest and boosted his confidence. A rejuvenated Elijah then rose up to defeat King Ahab and Jezebel.

God has promised: He will never leave or forsake us (Hebrews 13:5). He's never disengaged or distant, even if it feels like He is miles away. We need to develop the ability to practice His presence, especially during dark times. Don't let unreliable emotions dictate your response to trials or setbacks. Allow the certainty of His Presence to soak deep into your being, penetrating every thought and emotion. God delights in trumping appearances, and with Him close by, it's never as dark as it appears.

Lord, thank You that we can feel, even the feeling of sadness,
but wipe away our tears so that we will see Your presence in the midst of hard times.

Path to Peace

joe fornear

These things I have spoken to you, so that in Me you may have peace.
In the world you have tribulation, but take courage; I have overcome the world.

John 16:33

When you're suffering greatly, as so many of you are, inner peace is hard to find. Yet among His last words and testimony, Jesus provided a path to peace.

First, the peace we want and need is *in* Him, literally. John 14:27 says, "My peace I give to you." The peace He offers is the very peace He experiences inside of Himself. He has a secure and restful control over the universe. Do you think He frets or worries about the future? Never! He does not panic when things are tough. When we cling to Him for peace, He transfers His own calm assurance to us. It's a supernatural but simple process.

Next, realize that peace does not come because He removes our troubles. Some teach that if only we have enough faith, God will grant us trouble-free existence. Wrong. We must never fall into the trap of thinking our peace is dependent on our circumstances. He is crystal clear that He will *not* remove all hardships: "In this world you have tribulation." Still His promise remains: "the peace of God which surpasses understanding will guard our hearts and minds in Christ Jesus" (Philippians 4:7).

This peace, God's peace, "surpasses understanding." This means it doesn't make sense from a human standpoint. Harsh circumstances may rage around us, even within us in our bodies, yet we can remain calm and serene. Church history is full of stories of Christ-seekers who were tortured, even martyred, while simultaneously displaying a miraculous calm. They did it with His peace, and we can too.

Finally, He tells us in John 16:33 to "take courage." Some Bible versions translate this phrase "be of good cheer." How can we be of good cheer when our world is falling apart? By realizing He has ultimate control. "He has overcome the world!" He overcame by enduring the pain and storms of this world with poise and grace, and we can too—but only through Him.

Eventually He will enforce His absolute dominance over the universe. One day, He will remove every hardship. Revelation 21:4 proclaims, "He will wipe away every tear from their eyes; and there will no longer be any death; there will no longer be any mourning, or crying, or pain." The wonderful news is suffering and tribulations are temporary. So take courage and cheer up!

Let's stop trying to generate our own peace, or trying to find it in this world. His peace is free, it is beyond circumstances, and it works!

Lord, help us not try to manufacture peace, but rather draw from Your very own peace.

Three Doctrines to Buoy the Spirit and Anchor the Soul

joe fornear

In the same way God, desiring even more to show to the heirs of the promise the unchangeableness of His purpose, interposed with an oath, so that by two unchangeable things in which it is impossible for God to lie, we who have taken refuge would have strong encouragement to take hold of the hope set before us. This hope we have as an anchor of the soul, a hope both sure and steadfast.

Hebrews 6:17-19

It's great to know when we turn to the Lord, He promises to show up! Nothing makes Bible doctrine come to life like real-life desperation. While I was fighting cancer and being pummeled by discouraging thoughts, I was reassured by three unchangeable truths about the Lord that buoyed my spirit and anchored my soul.

The Sovereignty of God. Despite my pain, oppression and confusion, it was comforting to know He was still in absolute control over my life. Nothing is or can be stronger than Him. Nothing can stand in His way. Though medicine was proving powerless over the Stage IV metastatic melanoma which ravaged my pancreas, lung, kidney, stomach and lymph system, I knew God could remove every trace of cancer with a snap of His finger. He would have the last word, because He always has the last word. Jesus expressed the sovereignty of God in this way, "The things that are impossible with people are possible with God" (Luke 18:27). Does this truth lift your spirit?

The Goodness of God. God is good all of the time. He proved this forever when He sent His Son, Jesus Christ, to die for me while I was a sinner and His enemy (Romans 5:6–8). After adopting me as His son, how much more would He cause His goodness to spontaneously flow to me? Paul summarized the goodness of God in this way, "We know that God causes all things to work together for good to those who love God, to those who are called according to His purpose" (Romans 8:28). He pours out His goodness, enabling us to conquer anything.

The Incomprehensibility of God. Incomprehensibility is a big word, but the meaning is simple. There is much we don't understand about His ways. Asaph, the Psalmist, described His incomprehensibility in this way, "Your way was in the sea and Your paths in the mighty waters, and Your footprints may not be known" (Psalm 77:19). As with Israel at the Red Sea, God may carry us to a place that confuses and upsets us. We don't always see the way out, and He doesn't always explain why He allows painful seasons in our lives. But we don't have to trust blindly. We can be so certain of His sovereignty and goodness that we don't need to figure everything out! This lifts a heavy burden from us. We allow Him to navigate while we focus on enjoying the ride!

These three truths work together to provide a supernatural peace and stability no matter what happens.

Lord, when we don't understand what You are doing,
help us anchor our souls in Your loving control and care of our lives.

Holy Emotions

joe fornear

In the days of His flesh, He offered up both prayers and supplications with loud crying and tears to the One able to save Him from death, and He was heard because of His piety.

Hebrews 5:7

If Jesus displayed this type of raw emotion in a prayer meeting today, how do you think people would respond? Would He be taken aside and hushed? Would He be asked to find another prayer group? Some might consider His "loud crying and tears" as distracting at best, or perhaps even insensitive and rude. Others might "discern" that Jesus was trying to draw attention to Himself. Yet would anyone claim that Jesus was not "in the Spirit" when He prayed in this manner?

In the Garden of Gethsemane, on the night before He went to the cross, Jesus' prayer was so intense that He began to sweat blood. He was beyond upset. He was in deep distress and not afraid to let it out. "And being in agony He was praying very fervently; and His sweat became like drops of blood, falling down upon the ground" (Luke 22:44). So we should not be afraid to cry out to God in the midst of our crisis.

Evidently in Jesus Christ, the flame of God was stoked by powerful, earnest emotions. Yet it chills me to know that I could be so proper and distinguished that I extinguish the very fire of God in myself or others. Perhaps we are feeling so oppressed and depressed because we are suppressing valid emotions that should be poured out to God. I'm not suggesting these emotions must be publicly released, but don't be afraid to cry out to God in the midst of your crisis.

Lord, help us be real and allow ourselves to truly feel the intensity of our situations.
Help us pour out our hearts to You.

Time Out: Worry and Anxiety

terri fornear

*Look at the birds of the air; they do not sow or reap or store away in barns, and yet your heavenly
Father feeds them. Are you not much more valuable than they? Who of you by worrying can
add a single hour to his life? And why do you worry about clothes? See how the lilies of the field grow.
They do not labor or spin. Yet I tell you that not even Solomon in all his splendor was dressed
like one of these. If that is how God clothes the grass of the field, which is here today and tomorrow
is thrown into the fire, will he not much more clothe you, O you of little faith?*

Matthew 6:26-28

So much of life is timed. Work time, dinnertime, nighttime, vacation time, Christmastime, prayer time, etc. I'm either looking forward to something in the future, or remembering something about the past. Recently, I've been reading about the "Holiness of the Present Moment." I want to be walking in the NOW of life. When I do, life is so much lighter.

When I worry, a minute seems a lot longer than 60 seconds. Time slows down, and I grow more tired and worn out. Jesus talks about this in Matthew 6. He wants us to see and feel His love, so He invites us to consider the world around us. He says, look at the birds; look at the lilies. These are His creations, which we had nothing to do with creating or maintaining. They don't fret or worry. They are His work, completely cared for by Him. So since we are His most precious creations, the last thing we need to do is to worry.

The Holiness of the Present Moment is staying in each moment and looking to Him. This sets time apart from the tick of the clock to the awareness of His Presence at all times in all things. His reality and love are stronger than anything time brings.

♡

*Lord, help us fully trust that You are with us NOW,
and that You will never leave us to provide or fend for ourselves.*

Depression and Cancer

joe fornear

No temptation has overtaken you but such as is common to man; and God is faithful,
who will not allow you to be tempted beyond what you are able, but with the temptation
will provide the way of escape also, so that you will be able to endure it.

1 Corinthians 10:3

In our work with cancer patients, we are often asked the same question: "How can you deal with the depression this illness causes?" Depression is common with cancer, but as this verse in 1 Corinthians assures us, the Lord never gives us more than we can handle. We can say no to the temptation to be overwhelmed. So based on observing other patients, and dealing with my own depression during my cancer fight, I've compiled some steps that provide a way of escape from depression.

Give yourself a break. Many cancer patients beat themselves up for feeling down, which only makes them feel worse. I know this from personal experience. Cancer causes such high stress levels. When we consider all the elements of battling cancer, we find a perfect storm for depression. There are chain reaction struggles that form a vicious cycle. First the pain; then pain pills; then constipation from the pain pills; then enemas for the constipation; then hemorrhoids from the enemas; then pain from the hemorrhoids; then repeat. Chemotherapy can be an emotional depth charge—the vomiting, hair loss, weight loss and looking at the ashen, emaciated face in the mirror. No wonder we get depressed! It is natural to feel sad. If you don't feel sad when battling cancer, I would say that is a sign of emotional unhealthiness. So cut yourself some slack. It is natural to struggle.

Turn to the Lord and pour up your feelings to Him. Both Job and King David demonstrated symptoms of depression, including sleeplessness, constant tears, wanting to die and hopelessness. Interestingly, David was called "a man after God's own heart" (1 Samuel 13:14), yet neither he nor Job buried what they felt. They expressed their anguish and honestly placed their emotions before God.

God loves to show Himself in the midst of our pain and struggles. Your tendency might be to turn or drift away from the Lord, but even if you feel angry, actively turn toward Him instead. He can handle it. Be certain to ask Him for a response to your feelings, and then listen—He speaks in many different ways.

Talk to people who understand and ask for support. Find a support group, phone partner, crisis counselor or call us at Stronghold Ministry (see Appendix III for contact information). Depression can make us feel isolated and alone. You might be surprised how effectively others can help lighten your load. Don't be too proud to ask for help. Then, don't be afraid to ask someone who really encouraged you for more time together. If you think someone's presence would help you, risk letting them know. "Would you be open to visit me again? I really enjoyed spending time with you." Or, ask someone to read the Bible or a good book to you. Taking care of yourself entails asking for what you need.

Find an antidepressant that works for you. In general, I am not a strong proponent of antidepressant drugs. But since I was taking such powerful cancer drugs that induced depression, it made sense to me to try to balance my chemical system. The drug which worked best for me was Ativan, also called lorazepam, but keep experimenting with your doctor until you find one that works well for you. Unless you are an emotional mess in their office, not many oncologists probe for cancer-related depression. So if you seem to be coping well on the outside, you will probably need to ask your doctor for a prescription. Don't hesitate!

Make sense of your struggle. To help make sense of suffering and trials and to get an eternal perspective on their purpose, we strongly recommend a devotional book titled *Streams in the Desert*. This book helped me see God's higher purposes in my suffering. He is not a masochist in the sky, delighting in our suffering; nor is He ignoring our plight. He is good—all of the time, so take the time to learn more about His ways.

*Lord, fighting cancer has been overwhelming at times, but always remind us
that You never give more than we can handle, and You always provide a way of escape.*

Replacing Fear

terri fornear

We are destroying speculations and every lofty thing raised up against the knowledge of God, and we are taking every thought captive to the obedience of Christ.

2 Corinthians 10:5

I can so identify with the daily flow of e-mails and phone calls that come in to Stronghold Ministry. There is a certain fear that creeps in when a doctor first places that label of "cancer" on you. I remember our doctor sitting me down after Joe had some lymph nodes removed and tested. He told me it was "metastatic cancer." At first, I was thinking, *what kind of cancer is that?* I had not seen a lot of cancer in my family. So I just sat there, totally numb, with much fear of the unknown.

This was a time when an "intruder" came into my life. Bigger and stronger than me, I was taken off guard and paralyzed. It was a place where I felt totally alone and not equipped to win. I sometimes still face that feeling, yet it's in that place of fear that I am beginning to listen, really listen, to Another's voice.

I must replace the fears with His words. How many times did Jesus come to people and say, "Do not fear, I am here"? "Fear not, I will never leave you." He is so aware that we are fearful. He does not condemn us. He does not wait until we get our fear under control. No, He comes right into the midst of it, and says, "I AM here." Yes, He is right there with us in the middle of a fight with cancer.

What looks like the end is really the beginning of His love working deliverance. 1 John 4:18 says, "There is no fear in love; but perfect love casts out fear, because fear involves punishment, and the one who fears is not perfected in love." He is standing up against the fear in our lives and casting it out, while He perfects us in His love. He is not punishing us! He wants to use the "intruder" to bring in His unconditional love and grace to us and all those around us.

So what do we say to those who call or write us about their fears with cancer? I stand with them and Jesus, casting out fear with His perfect love. This is how

Stronghold Ministry gives people the message of Jesus' abundant grace, and shares His gift of righteousness to all that receive Him.

Lord, we want to be controlled by Your love, not fear, so we come against the lie of fear and declare Your presence and protection over our lives.

Disappointment with God

joe fornear

Now when John, while imprisoned, heard of the works of Christ, he sent word by his disciples and said to Him, "Are You the Expected One, or shall we look for someone else?"

Matthew 11:2-3

The Bible is filled with stories of people who were deeply disappointed with God's path for their lives. Consider John the Baptist, who had been imprisoned for his penetrating preaching. He had done nothing wrong. In fact, it was his faithfulness in holding up God's standards that had landed him in jail. No doubt he was expecting Jesus to free him quickly. He was, after all, Jesus' "right hand man." The prophets had not only foretold Jesus' coming, but John's coming as well! It was right there in Isaiah! John was "the voice" sent to prepare the way of the Lord. And so he waited.

As the days slipped by and he heard more and more reports about Jesus' miracles, John's frustration grew. At first glance, the question he relayed to Jesus might appear innocent, but his exasperation spills out. "Shall we look for someone else?" Surely the Messiah would deliver his cousin, friend and the one who had introduced him to the world. So perhaps Jesus was not who he claimed to be? I don't think John ever doubted Jesus' identity, but he certainly questioned Jesus' judgment. Jesus' response seems to confirm that John was indeed deeply disillusioned with Him: "Blessed is he who does not stumble over me." John's appeal was designed to prod Jesus into springing him from jail, yet Jesus never answered that prayer. God had a higher purpose in taking John home to heaven.

How then do we manage our expectations so we don't slip into despair? I think we must realize Jesus promised freedom in the midst of trials—not freedom from trials. In John 16:33, Jesus assures us, "These things I have spoken to you, so that in Me you may have peace. In the world you have tribulation, but take courage; I have overcome the world."

On the night before His trek to the cross, even Jesus struggled with God's plan for His life. He sought three times for His Father to change the plan, but the Father did not budge. Jesus found hope in the Father's promise of joy after suffering. "So fixing our eyes on Jesus, the author and perfecter of faith, who for the joy set before Him endured the cross, despising the shame, and has sat down at the right hand of the throne of God" (Hebrews 12:2). Even though we don't always understand the Father's mind, we can always trust His heart.

Lord, we admit we are sometimes disillusioned by Your plan for our lives,
but help us focus on the joy in submitting to Your plan.

Tear Collector

joe fornear

Every night I make my bed swim, I dissolve my couch with my tears.

Psalm 6:6

God has allowed some of His closest servants to suffer greatly. David was a magnet for suffering, attracting multitudes of enemies. Like a wild game animal, David was hunted across the wilderness by Saul, whom God had permitted to usurp David's throne. As David hid, he was often forced into the hate-filled Philistine's territory. His soul had no rest from valid fears. It wasn't his imagination; many plotted his demise and death. He often found himself exhausted and alone in the wilderness.

David's memoirs in the Psalms reveal the depths of his distress and describe the sheer volume of tears from a man who killed lions and bears—and Goliath, the giant. Evidently, real men do cry. "Every night I make my bed swim, I dissolve my couch with my tears" (Psalm 6:6). Did God notice David's tears? Does God care about our tears?

"You have taken account of my wanderings. Put my tears in Your bottle. Are they not in Your book?" (Psalm 56:8). God considers tears to be liquid prayers. This verse says He not only notices our tears, He collects them. Like people collect stamps or coins, God keeps a book with pages stained by your tears. He knows the journeys of those who wander in the wilderness in the enemy territory of cancer. He is noticing, watching, tracking each step and bottling our tears.

God is always for you, whether you're wandering in the wilderness, or fighting for your life. So, like David, say to yourself, "This I know, that God is for me." (Psalm 56:9).

♡

Lord, we thank You for not only noticing our tears but sitting with us to comfort us in our distress.

Where Is God When It Hurts?

joe fornear

In all their affliction He was afflicted, and the angel of His presence saved them. In His love and in His mercy He redeemed them, and He lifted them and carried them all the days of old.

Isaiah 63:9

Where is God when it hurts? During a cancer battle, some may not ask this question, but I did during my battle. I really wanted to know the answer. Isaiah provides a glimpse into unseen realities. God is not only present and watching, He is actually hurting too! "In all their affliction He was afflicted." In addition, He "lifts us and carries us" through the entire trial. This truly shows His "love and mercy" for us.

This shouldn't surprise us. The Lord instructs us in Romans 12:15 to "weep with those who weep." Since He never asks us to care in ways that He doesn't, it follows that He weeps along with us. For example, recall John 11 when Lazarus died. His sisters, Mary and Martha, were soaked with tears. Jesus knew this story would have a happy ending. In just minutes, after Lazarus was resurrected, uncontrollable joy would fill each grief-filled heart. Still John 11:35 tells us that "Jesus wept." So why in the world would He cry at that moment? I think He so identifies with our pain that He cannot help but to hurt when we are hurting. What an awesome God we have the privilege of knowing and serving!

In addition, recall when Paul, then called Saul, was en route to persecute Jesus' followers again. Jesus suddenly appeared, blinding Saul and knocking him off his high horse. In a voice that resembled a thunder clap, Jesus challenged him, "Why are you persecuting *Me*?" Jesus took Paul's attacks on His beloved children quite personally. Again, He hurts when we hurt.

Jesus also explained that when we visit and help those who are sick or imprisoned, they help and visit *Him*. "Truly I say to you, to the extent that you did it to one of these brothers of Mine, even the least of them, you did it to Me" (Matthew 25:40). He truly identifies with us in our suffering.

So now we know exactly where God is when we hurt. He is right beside us, feeling our pain and carrying us through every trial! This lightens my load. How about you?

Thank You, Lord, for your incredibly caring heart toward us, Your children.

SUFFERING

Is God Up To Something?

joe fornear

For I consider that the sufferings of this present time are not worthy to be compared with the glory that is to be revealed to us.

Romans 8:18

Was God up to something when He allowed Joseph to be sold into slavery by his own brothers, left to rot in prison and then falsely accused of rape? Yes! God used these pain-filled events to maneuver Joseph into prominence in Egypt, a position from which Joseph "saved" the lives of his brothers and his father, Jacob. Joseph's suffering was worth it in the end.

Was God up to something when He allowed Job to lose his possessions, children and his health? Yes! The book of Job has provided comfort to hundreds of millions, perhaps billions of sufferers. Job's suffering was worth it in the end.

Was God up to something when He allowed Paul to be imprisoned for sharing the good news of Jesus Christ? Yes! Ironically, it was from prison that Paul wrote the tremendously freeing epistles of Ephesians, Colossians and Philippians. Paul's suffering was worth it in the end.

Was God up to something when He allowed the deaths of Naomi's husband and two sons? Yes! God used Naomi's daughter-in-law, Ruth, who followed her back from Moab, to be in the lineage of not only King David but also of Jesus Christ. Naomi's suffering was worth it in the end.

Did these heroes and heroines always know what God was up to? No! Most had no clue of the manner in which God was about to use their troubles.

Is God up to something in *your* sufferings and mine? Definitely! Our suffering will be worth it in the end. Yet what if our sufferings do not result in such a spectacular outcome? If we can bring one bit of glory to God through our sufferings, it will be worth it in the end. His glory far outshines our sufferings.

Lord, we now see dimly through the fog of our cancer battles,
yet grant us that deep certainty that you are indeed up to something good.

Is Pain In Vain?

joe fornear

My thoughts are not your thoughts, and My ways are not your ways.

Isaiah 55:9

I have a belief that might make some cringe: There were benefits to my battle with cancer. Now before you conclude I'm losing my grip, let's remember God works in ways that may seem contradictory to us. He acknowledges the oddity of *our* ways, "My thoughts are not your thoughts, and My ways are not your ways" (Isaiah 55:9).

William Cowper composed a hymn with this theme, "God works in mysterious ways, His wonders to perform." Later in the song, a provocative line captures God's positive leveraging of suffering: "The bud may have a bitter taste, but sweet will be the flower."

It doesn't appear that Paul, the suffering apostle, had cancer, but he was definitely acquainted with pain, as 2 Corinthians 11:23–25 makes clear.

[I have been] in far more labors, in far more imprisonments, beaten times without number, often in danger of death. Five times I received from the Jews thirty-nine lashes. Three times I was beaten with rods, once I was stoned, three times I was shipwrecked, a night and a day I have spent in the deep.

Paul had been physically battered by enemies of Christ because of his loyalty to God. He knew how to cope with the emotional and physical turmoil. One might say he was an expert in pain management. In 2 Corinthians 4:16–18, he stressed a valuable benefit of suffering which helped him get through the horrible treatment he received.

Therefore we do not lose heart, but though our outer man is decaying, yet our inner man is being renewed day by day. For momentary, light affliction is producing for us an eternal weight of glory far beyond all comparison, while we look not at the things which are seen, but at the things which are not seen; for the things which are seen are temporal, but the things which are not seen are eternal.

If physical pain is correctly leveraged, it sets us free from temporal, tangible things, and redirects us to eternal, unseen things. In other words, the comforts of this life will not distract us from eternal realities. Let's face it—this earth is not our final destination. We can become so caught up in earthly niceties—like homes, cars, vacations, experiences and accomplishments. No matter how many times He heals us in this life, we must eventually abandon the things of this world. So suffering, though unpleasant, performs a valuable function.

During my cancer battle, I constantly grieved that I could not play basketball or go fishing. Though I really enjoyed these activities, I discovered I could live without them. Don't get me wrong, God delights in giving us good things here on this earth, but there is a difference between enjoying things and being entangled by them. Battling cancer helped me grasp the difference. I still have a long way to go, but my grip on an eternal perspective is now more firm.

Let's not waste our suffering. Let it become a portal for God's best for us.

Lord, help us grasp the powerful and freeing lessons You teach us through suffering and pain.

Now That's Hard

joe fornear

Beloved, do not be surprised at the fiery ordeal among you, which comes upon you for your testing, as though some strange thing were happening to you; but to the degree that you share the sufferings of Christ, keep on rejoicing, so that also at the revelation of His glory you may rejoice with exultation.

1 Peter 4:12–13

There was a story that first appeared in a newspaper in Galveston, Texas, about a woman and her parakeet named Chippie. One day Chippie was flying happily around his cage, until his owner got the bright idea to tidy up his cage with a vacuum cleaner. You know what's coming—when the phone rang, she left the vacuum nozzle wedged into the cage and "ffwhompp," little Chippie took the ride of his life. His owner quickly dug him out of the dust bag. He was blanketed with dust, so she thrust him under running water for a while. He started shivering, so he was introduced to the high heat setting of the hair dryer. Is anyone surprised that since the ordeal, his owner reports, "Chippie doesn't sing much anymore. He just sits and stares"?

Have you been under trials that seem to have buried you? Have you lost your song? Satan would have you believe that you have been singled out for hardship. Why me, Lord? But God wants us to fight off despair and self-pity. He says through Peter, "Resist Satan, firm in your faith, knowing that the same experiences of suffering are being accomplished by your brethren who are in the world" (1 Peter 5:9).

I recently discovered a provocative book about the sufferings Christian people have been experiencing around the world. Christians in Sudan have been raped, others pillaged, and two million have been killed for their faith. In light of these revelations, permit me to paraphrase 1 Peter 5:9, "Stand firm against Satan, and resist complaining, because compared to many Christians in the world, your lives are rather easy."

News from Sudan includes the humbling report that the favorite verse of many of the persecuted Christians is 2 Corinthians 4:17–18, "For momentary, light affliction is producing for us an eternal weight of glory far beyond all comparison, while we look not at the things which are seen, but at the things which are not seen; for the things which are seen are temporal, but the things which are not seen are eternal." *Light* afflictions?!

Oh Lord, deliver us from self-absorption and give us the zeal
to serve You and persevere through our trials.

Did God Punish Me With Cancer?

joe fornear

As He passed by, He saw a man blind from birth. And His disciples asked Him, "Rabbi, who sinned, this man or his parents, that he would be born blind?" Jesus answered, "It was neither that this man sinned, nor his parents; but it was so that the works of God might be displayed in him."

John 9:1-3

The notion that bad things happen to bad people is rooted deep in the thinking of mankind. It was prevalent in Job's time as his "friends" heaped accusations on him. To them, Job had obviously sinned to deserve such horrific circumstances.

Despite the clarity of the book of Job that God disconnected trouble and His punishment, the thinking persisted into Jesus' time in the first century. The situation in John 9 presented a dilemma for this mind-set. If a person was *born* with a disability such as blindness, could that mean God was punishing the parent's sin? Just as Yahweh rebuked Job's friends, Jesus rebuked His disciples for their judgmental attitudes. Jesus said the man was born blind so that Jesus could heal Him and display His Father's glory and power. Human suffering may have nothing to do with divine punishment!

Even today cancer patients ask us if perhaps God gave them cancer to punish them. While certainly God uses cancer as a wake-up call to secure our attention, His punishment is reserved for the afterlife. His goal in our lives today is to save us, not punish us. Jesus told His bloodthirsty disciples who wanted Him to annihilate the Samaritans, "You do not know what kind of spirit you are of, for the Son of Man did not come to destroy men's lives, but to save them" (Luke 9:56).

You see, Jesus Christ stepped in to take man's punishment for sin upon Himself. This is precisely why Jesus died. God is not, therefore, punishing us with cancer.

I don't want to misrepresent the need for repentance and our accountability before God. Jesus warns that divine punishment will ultimately come if a person does not repent. Yet repentance and faith in Him is all He requires.

Now on the same occasion there were some present who reported to Him about the Galileans whose blood Pilate had mixed with their sacrifices. And Jesus said to them, "Do you suppose that these Galileans were greater sinners than all other Galileans because they suffered this fate? I tell you, no, but unless you repent, you will all likewise perish. Or do you suppose that those eighteen on whom the tower in Siloam fell and killed them were worse culprits than all the men who live in Jerusalem? I tell you, no, but unless you repent, you will all likewise perish" (Luke 13:1–5).

The word "repentance" means literally "to change one's mind." We must be convinced that we have sinned and that we need forgiveness. Then we are primed to receive the *free* gift of forgiveness and righteousness through receiving Christ as our personal Savior. Find out more about receiving Christ as Savior by reading "The Two Ways to Get to Heaven" (Appendix II).

I believe God delights in showing off His grace. Paul the apostle and King David were especially anointed by God to speak on His behalf. They both confessed their sin, and testified that God does not punish us for sins which He has forgiven. In Romans 4:7–8, Paul quotes David in Psalm 32:1–2, "Blessed are those whose lawless deeds have been forgiven, and whose sins have been covered. Blessed is the man whose sin the Lord will not take into account."

I suspect Paul and David were both relieved to experience God's gracious forgiveness, because both men committed murder! As such, they would have been prime candidates for being immediately and severely punished by God. Think about it—how blessed we are when the Lord passes over our sin!

Lord, open our eyes to see the extent of Your grace and mercy to us because of Jesus Christ.

The Great Consolation

joe fornear

That I may know Him and the power of His resurrection and the fellowship of His sufferings.

Philippians 3:10

We seek to console people who are experiencing considerable pain. When pain wracks the body, it seizes the attention of our entire being. We cry out for relief to God and man. When relief is not found or granted, what then? Could there be some redeeming benefit to pain and suffering?

Like us, Paul sought God to remove his painful trials. Paul certainly understood pain. A partial list of his sufferings is found in 2 Corinthians 12:24–25, "Five times I received from the Jews thirty-nine lashes. Three times I was beaten with rods, once I was stoned." When release from these sufferings did not come, he discovered The Great Consolation, knowing Jesus Christ, the great soother of pain.

For Paul, having a tight relationship with Jesus became the overriding goal of his life. Pain relief was secondary. But why? What did he gain from knowing Christ?

Paul provides several points of gain in knowing Christ through pain:

Knowing Him is the ultimate discovery of life! "I count all things to be loss in view of the surpassing value of knowing Christ Jesus my Lord" (Philippians 3: 8). Paul reset his affections from lesser, worldly desires, to what he saw as the ultimate treasure, Jesus Christ. As a result, he experienced incredible kindness, love and comfort from Christ. Thus he was drawn deeper and deeper into experiencing the most attractive Being in the universe. Could pain be the unexpected catalyst to awaken you to life's most rewarding relationship?

Sharing in His sufferings leads to sharing in His resurrection power. In Philippians 3:10, Paul says his goal is "That I may know Him and the power of His resurrection and the fellowship of His sufferings" (Philippians 3:10).

When we turn to Him in our pain, He touches us with His powerful presence. His resurrection power surges into and through us. His strength is perfected in our weakness. We find ourselves in His grip with an "other-worldly" peace and unquenchable hope.

We gain clarity of purpose to focus on pursuing eternal goals. "I press on toward the goal for the prize of the upward call of God in Christ Jesus" (Philippians 3:14). In other words, it is extremely wise to leverage our time and efforts for eternally rewarding purposes. Then in the end, the payoff will be crystal clear. We will have answered His call, and thereby stored up vast treasures in heaven! This is the ultimate focus, to tell of His goodness in every circumstance.

When we take our suffering and pain to the Lord, He pulls back the curtain to show us Himself. He is The Great Consolation. Where are you turning in the midst of your pain? Let's draw near to Him—*through* the pain.

Lord, use our pain to draw us from the things of this world into Your Presence, power and purposes.

PRAISE

♡

Thankful In Everything?

joe fornear

In everything give thanks; for this is God's will for you in Christ Jesus.
1 Thessalonians 5:18

Sometimes God's requests seem illogical, sometimes impossible and sometimes both. How can we give thanks in the midst of excruciating pain or overwhelming grief? This is precisely, however, what He asks, and Paul seems to anticipate resistance. He adds, "This is His will for you in Christ Jesus."

It may be *His* will for us to give thanks in everything, but is it *our* will? Honestly, during my battle with cancer, thankfulness was not often on my radar screen. But if a loving God wants us to do something, it must somehow benefit us, even if we don't understand how. Once we shift over to thanksgiving, we discover the Lord's wisdom, as perspective changes everything.

So thankfulness makes sense, but is it always possible? Job proved humans can give thanks despite great grief and pain. He praised and worshiped God after the death of his children, servants and livestock. Then he blessed God despite an incredibly painful skin disease.

We can imitate Job because we have the same resources from which to draw. In fact, in this New Testament era, we have more resources than Job since Jesus Christ's supernatural power and inheritance is available to us.

So giving thanks in every situation is not only logical, but possible. The following are three points for which I was especially thankful during my battle.

God's nearness. He revealed His presence to me in tangible ways. More than once He gave me a peace which could not be explained, especially given my physical and emotional condition. It certainly didn't come from me!

People's support. Though people could not take away my suffering, they surely lightened my load. I was often amazed and thankful for the genuine care I received from so many, even total strangers! Another's love should never be taken for granted.

Clearer perspective. Being incapacitated revealed the shallowness of some of my normal pursuits. One example: I "saw" the emptiness of popular culture. Or did I see my own emptiness, to be so mindlessly entertained and distracted by so little?

Lord, we hurt, still help us to focus on the many things for which we can be thankful.

Acing Your Tests

joe fornear

Consider it all joy, my brethren, when you encounter various trials,
knowing that the testing of your faith produces endurance.

James 1:2-3

I like to watch kids at the end of the school year. Naturally, they have an extra bounce in their step. Were you ever sorry when school was out for the summer? No more classes, homework or *tests*? For me it was easy to trade tests for fishing, playing ball and riding my bike. Yet James asks mature adults to have a different perspective on tests. We are to "consider it all joy" when our faith is tested.

Tests of faith may reveal how little we know of the subject matter. Tests can be painful as well, and their timing is never convenient. Some people may be disturbed by James' view of tests, such as in the case of natural catastrophes—or cancer. Is it even possible to count it all joy when your eyes are filled with tears? Can we have a positive attitude as our world seems to crumble at our feet? Can joy exist in the soul when the body is wracked with pain of chemo or tumors, or both? James believes it's possible because God can help us "pass" these tests.

James teaches that trials have a straightforward goal: endurance. Why endurance? Consider children, their immaturity is expressed in constant need to be entertained and in their intolerance of adversity. Mature adults accept and patiently work through hard times and their character becomes fully developed. They are truly happy, as circumstances don't dictate their moods.

Thank God, a permanent break from tests will come at our ultimate graduation into heaven. In the meantime, we are not left to our own resources to pass these tests. The Lord provides supernatural strength so we can patiently bear the unbearable. This is how we "Let endurance have its perfect work, so that we may be perfect and complete, lacking in nothing" (James 1:4).

Fortunately, the Lord allows us to see the correct answers during our tests of faith. He gives wisdom to lead us through the confusion (James 1:5–8). Our teacher is the tested, tried and true one, Jesus Christ, who is indeed "the author and perfecter of our faith" (Hebrews 12:2). He offers unlimited retakes of our tests, which is a very good thing for me. How about you?

Lord, we want to grow in character by patiently and joyfully enduring hard times.

Giving Thanks During a Crisis

joe fornear

*Be anxious for nothing, but in everything by prayer and supplication with thanksgiving
let your requests be made known to God.*

Philippians 4:6

Crisis often brings a new closeness to God. When fighting for survival, even hard core do-it-yourselfers turn to the One who can do anything. If you're like me, this closeness often takes the form of prayer requests, asking Him to intervene. Now, don't get me wrong, Jesus delighted in bold requests for miraculous intervention. We all would like harsh circumstances removed quickly. Jesus can certainly identify with us. He asked the Father for a Plan B, that the salvation of mankind might possibly come by some less painful means.

Yet God asks when we petition Him that we also give thanks. Sometimes the last thing we feel like doing is thanking God. Keep in mind the Lord anticipated such moments. In Psalm 50:23, He says, "He who offers a sacrifice of thanksgiving honors Me." As usual, God never asks or commands us to do anything that is not for our greatest good. He also provides the enablement to do His will in every situation.

The following are three encouraging reasons to mix thanks with our requests:

Thanksgiving transforms our outlook and mood. When we count our blessings accurately, we move beyond the old saying of seeing the cup half full or half empty; we'll have "eyes to see" that we have *many* full cups! We'll acknowledge and deeply appreciate the huge list of prayers He's already answered. We have food and clothing, love from people and modern luxuries filling our homes. Any one of these luxuries, such as a phone, makes us the envy of past generations. These are all His gifts and should not be taken for granted.

Thanksgiving builds contentment into our character. Character is what separates an unhappy, spoiled child from a happy, well-adjusted child. One child frets over what he does not have; the other enjoys what he does have. Contentment frees up adult children as well. I admit many times during my battle with Stage IV metastatic melanoma, I was neither thankful nor content. But Christ gave me strength to get back on track, no matter what was happening. Paul said in Philippians 4:11 and 13, "I have learned to be content in whatever circumstances I am. I can do all things through Him who strengthens me." Contentment is an incredible gift!

Thanksgiving keeps us alert to unseen blessings. "Devote yourselves to prayer, keeping alert in it with thanksgiving" (Colossians 4:2). While we ask for earthly blessings, an attitude of thanksgiving keeps us alert to the many ways the Lord has spiritually provided. We have an amazing bundle of riches from God that come to us freely in Christ. These include love, joy, peace, forgiveness and eternal salvation. The promise of the free gift of eternal salvation is enough motivation to be forever thankful, even if God never gives us another thing in this life! Being attuned and thankful for spiritual realities lifts us above our temporary earthly afflictions.

Lord, adjust our focus so that we want to give thanks in crisis and out of crisis.

Hope
amy fornear

And we exult in hope of the glory of God. And not only this, but we also exult in our tribulations, knowing that tribulation brings about perseverance; and perseverance, proven character; and proven character, hope; and hope does not disappoint, because the love of God has been poured out within our hearts through the Holy Spirit who was given to us.

Romans 5:2-5

(Amy is Joe and Terri's daughter. She wrote this poem in 2003 when she was 16 years old.
Joe's cancer at this time had spread to 13 different sites.)

Hope is what you need
When you've
Stepped the last step,
Raced the last race,
Swam the last meter.

It's when you see struggles
And the worst of life
In a different perspective
Than those who have views of despair.

Lord, help us never give up hope, even when things look so bleak.

Praising Through Pain

joe fornear

In this you greatly rejoice, even though now for a little while, if necessary, you have been distressed by various trials, so that the proof of your faith, being more precious than gold which is perishable, even though tested by fire, may be found to result in praise and glory and honor at the revelation of Jesus Christ; and though you have not seen Him, you love Him, and though you do not see Him now, but believe in Him, you greatly rejoice with joy inexpressible and full of glory.

1 Peter 1:6-8

These verses uncover the big picture connection of praise and suffering. If you're like me, worshipping God is easy when life is pleasant. Put me on a highway breezing along with the windows down and a good song on the radio and God and I are tight. But throw in a traffic jam and my zeal cools off considerably. When I face a bona fide test, like chronic pain, my appreciation for God seems to plummet. Difficult circumstances force us all to decide: is praise a reward we give God for His treating us favorably, or is praising Him unconditional?

Rejoicing while suffering is great theory, but how do we make it habit? How do I snap out of the doldrums? These verses from 1 Peter shed some helpful light.

Value the Lord more than the things of this world. Peter compares our faith to gold for a reason. Impurities in gold are burned off by fire, making it more genuine, shiny and valuable. In a similar way, the heat of suffering can clear out any impure dependence on human crutches, such as entertainment or material things. Knowing Christ's love is a windfall blessing if we turn to Him instead of the world's offerings. Peter connects the dots for us; if we don't suffer, we will not experience the depths of Christ's goodness. We can fight God about this, but He is clear that the path to great freedom in Christ usually entails pain.

Realize we are not the focus. One day we will truly grasp that the overall purpose of this universe was and is about God, not us. There will come a day when the only issue will be whether we honored Him during our brief lives here on earth. So what then is more important—His glory or my comfort?

Adopt a long-term, eternal perspective. Peter then emphasizes that at the end of time as we know it, the focal point of history will be revealed—the Lord Jesus Christ in all His glory. Suffering helps focus our priorities on His eternal purposes. We can become so distracted by temporary goals, such as bank accounts or popularity.

Praise Him anyway. We are taught early in life to thank people when they do something nice, and to avoid people who hurt us. So why in the world would we praise God when He allows persistent pain? When we truly grasp that suffering is rooted in God's best intentions for us, we will choose praise in spite of our circumstances. So praise Him always!

Lord, You are worth so much that it is a small thing to suffer to know You better.

STRENGTH
through
WEAKNESS

It's Supernatural

joe fornear

We have this treasure in earthen vessels, so that the surpassing greatness of the power
will be of God and not from ourselves.

2 Corinthians 4:7

At one point during my cancer fight in 2003, I finally acknowledged the battle was too much for me to bear alone. Believe me, I resisted the admission as long as I could. Early on, my mantra was: "Be strong, you can beat this." At age 44, I was relatively young, and in fairly good physical shape. I figured I was as prepared as anyone. I felt I could master the physical pain after years of pushing my body in sports and construction work. I could certainly handle the emotional stress because I was a tough guy from Pittsburgh, Pennsylvania, the Steel City of Champions. Plus I had been a pastor for 12 years, teaching others how to handle even the most difficult trials.

My natural strength held up well until the Stage IV metastatic melanoma spread beyond the lymph nodes under my arm to several internal organs. Three surgeries in a month, harsh chemo treatments and a steady barrage of complications took their toll. My illusions of strength faded to pleas for mercy. Like Peter sinking in the Sea of Galilee, I desperately reached out for help.

The Lord had been waiting all along, ready to lift me from the unstable sea of self-trust. Now years after recovering, the Lord must still continually remind me of my limitations. Perhaps my greatest deception is that I cling to wanting to be strong apart from Him. In Ephesians 6:10, Paul prods us past human power, "Be strong in the Lord and in the strength of *His* might." Fighting cancer and facing the hurdles of this life requires great strength. So why settle for natural strength, when we can tap the limitless, supernatural strength of Almighty God? He is our Stronghold! When we embrace our weakness, we experience His strength. So turn to Him for the all of the strength you need. He is waiting.

♡

Lord, break us from living out of our own strength, so that we live out of Your mighty power.

Such a Time As This

joe fornear

And who knows whether you have not attained royalty for such a time as this?

Esther 4:14

Would you believe there is an entire book of the Bible in which the name of God is never mentioned? It's true. God's name is not to be found in the book of Esther.

Why would such a book be included in the Bible? I believe the message is His work is often behind the scenes, even during devastating setbacks. Do you see the hand of God in the setbacks of your life? I admit, sometimes it is hard for me to "locate" Him when I am in pain. Frankly, sometimes I have a hard time finding Him when I am simply inconvenienced, like when something breaks around the house.

Esther's story was difficult from the beginning. She was orphaned and later forced to join a harem of a Persian king. Her Jewish nationality was about to be made public which at that time would have meant death, as the Jews were scheduled to be annihilated.

On the surface, God seemed absent, but was He? Esther's guardian Mordecai told her, "Perhaps you have been raised up for such a time as this." Mordecai was right. God used her connection to the king to save not only her life, but the entire Jewish nation. When God wants to show Himself and display His glory, He often begins in the midst of a crisis.

For millions of people the crisis through which God wants to reveals Himself is cancer. On the surface, being diagnosed may seem to be the mother of all setbacks. How can a loving, compassionate God be part of a cancer story? Though He may seem absent in our pain, He is always working behind the scenes toward a higher purpose.

I have come to view my own encounter with cancer as having a higher purpose. I think God raised me up, or rather laid me low, to help others understand Him better in the midst of their crisis. Cancer can be such a wake-up call.

It makes us pause to consider so many questions we had been taking for granted.

Could it be God has been working behind the scenes in your trials in order to display Himself in you and through you? Are you willing to suffer for His higher purposes?

Lord, we ask You to show us our setbacks in a whole new light—Your light.

Help!

joe fornear

For we do not have a high priest who cannot sympathize with our weaknesses, but One who has been tempted in all things as we are, yet without sin. Therefore let us draw near with confidence to the throne of grace, so that we may receive mercy and find grace to help in time of need.

Hebrews 4:15-16

Sometimes the concepts in these two verses get separated, and we forget their amazing connection. The One who now dispenses grace and mercy from the universe's throne once struggled with the same human weaknesses which we experience!

Jesus Christ suffered and then became the perfect liaison between God's resources and our needs. He was tested, and mastered every type of battle—physical, emotional, relational and spiritual. He did not seek out suffering. In fact, He sought to avoid the agony of the cross. He's felt the sting of man's rejection. He was misunderstood, judged and publicly humiliated. He knows what it's like to cry out to God, yet still feel forsaken.

So with hard-earned sympathy and empathy, Jesus offers His help, His grace. Grace is basically a supernatural ability to cope. He wants to be with us, and carry us through our battles. He is not some distant monarch, but a tender shepherd who guides us and strengthens us.

In addition to grace, this verse says He grants mercy. Unlike Jesus, I have not always handled suffering well. During my battle, I complained, raged and wallowed in self-pity. I was often frustrated that I could not handle the battle. Though He knew my sins and weaknesses, He continued to plead with me to draw near to Him. It was as if He were saying, "Don't let the past stop you from seeking My help now." This is mercy. He always forgives if we approach through Jesus Christ's work on the cross, not our own works.

In the end, His grace and mercy are "sufficient," enabling us to weather impossible circumstances. He took on our substantial weakness, so we could partake of His incredible strength. So boldly ask and expect Him to help in your time of need!

Lord, it is so comforting to know You experienced all of the hardship and temptations we face, and You offer to help us through them now.

Remember the Weakness
joe fornear

I am the vine, you are the branches; he who abides in Me and I in him, he bears much fruit, for apart from Me you can do nothing.

John 15:5

God is never helpless. He is never out of control. On the other hand, we are not in control, and from time to time, the Lord reminds us. I confess He must often go beyond simply reminding me to convincing me of my powerlessness. I tend to drift toward self-sufficiency and self-direction.

I wonder if one of my greatest sins is presumption. I fancy myself as able and competent, yet the Lord says everything we have is a gift. "What do you have that you did not receive?" (1 Corinthians 4:7). My ability to work hard, my talents, even my breath—all are gifts from God.

So I try to remember His lessons on powerlessness. I recall the "daymare," a nightmare which is not a dream. During those times of intense struggle, God showed me how utterly weak I was and am apart from Him. That sense of overwhelming weakness was very displeasing to my "can-do" ego. Jesus said in John 15:5 that we "can do *nothing* apart from Him."

My inability to cope on my own compelled me to cling to His strength, as mine was so quickly and totally expended. Paul says it best in 2 Corinthians 10:9, "And He has said to me, 'My grace is sufficient for you, for power is perfected in weakness.'"

It's easy to be a kind of "foxhole" Christian, so that we draw on God's strength only when we are under fire and desperate. Yet He desires that we be dependent on Him as a lifestyle, not just when we're in trouble. He continually reminds us of our weakness through circumstances that are "over our heads." 2 Corinthians 10:10 says, "Most gladly, therefore, I will rather boast about my weaknesses, so that the power of Christ may dwell in me. Therefore I am well content with weaknesses, with insults, with distresses, with persecutions, with difficulties, for Christ's sake; for when I am weak, then I am strong." Are you glad that you are weak?

♡

Lord, please keep us ever mindful of our weakness, as we want to be a channel for Your power.

Weak Link

joe fornear

Grace and peace be multiplied to you in the knowledge of God and of Jesus our Lord; seeing that His divine power has granted to us everything pertaining to life and godliness, through the true knowledge of Him who called us by His own glory and excellence. For by these He has granted to us His precious and magnificent promises, so that by them you may become partakers of the divine nature.

2 Peter 1:2-4

Weakness. It's been dismissed, denied and despised. Never let them see you sweat. Right? Wrong! We need to be honest and admit it—we are weak. Our personal strength is a straw hut against so many of the forces in this world. Can human determination stop a tornado from hitting a house? Can positive thinking keep the country's economy strong? Can mind over matter prevent serious illness from striking one's life? Does careful planning keep one's heart and lungs pumping overnight while sleeping? We are very weak.

Early in his relationship with Jesus, Peter was brimming with self-confidence. He would remain loyal and fight to his last breath, even if all the other disciples deserted Jesus. He thought he was in control. He believed he was strong in himself. Yet when his time to stand up for Jesus came, he shrunk back from the challenge. The experience humbled him. We might even say it humiliated him, and Peter was ready to give up.

Yet, Jesus was not done with him. Peter simply needed true humility, and to live out of the Holy Spirit's power, not his own. On the day of Pentecost, after he was filled with the Spirit, Peter was able to boldly proclaim the good news of Christ.

In the end, when Peter writes his second epistle, we can witness his amazing transformation. God opened his eyes to "see" the secret of living for the Lord. "Seeing that His divine power has granted to us everything pertaining to life and godliness" (2 Peter 1:3).

Lord, help us never be confident in ourselves, but only in Your power and life within us.

Trickle Down Love

joe fornear

But I thought it necessary to send to you Epaphroditus, my brother and fellow worker and fellow soldier, who is also your messenger and minister to my need; because he was longing for you all and was distressed because you had heard that he was sick. For indeed he was sick to the point of death, but God had mercy on him, and not on him only but also on me, so that I would not have sorrow upon sorrow. Therefore I have sent him all the more eagerly so that when you see him again you may rejoice and I may be less concerned about you.

Philippians 2:25-28

My father raised me to fear nothing. In his younger days, he was a successful running back in football, not the kind of running back that runs around people, but the kind that runs over people. He was a drill sergeant in the army—need I say more? He was always a can-do, nothing-can-stop-me-now guy. I did not have many opportunities to see his vulnerabilities or his soft side.

There was a time, however, when we almost lost my mom due to complications from surgery to remove some spots on her lungs that were cancerous. We knew there were risks to the operation, but she had gotten through invasive surgery before. We really weren't prepared for the attack of pneumonia that followed the surgery and the very serious four-day coma she experienced.

After she had pulled out of the coma, we were ecstatic and relieved. I was deeply touched by one of my dad's comments to me. He said, "The whole thing scared me to death." This may sound strange, but that piece of information still moves me today. I am sad my dad had to suffer during that time, but it struck me how much he loved my mom, and that gave me a real sense of security. I felt extra proud to be part of my family. We were a team, and each member was significant, especially the family members who started the whole thing. I'll never forget that glimpse of my dad's heart so many years ago.

One might think Paul never had any worries or fears for his friend's health, as he had a gift of performing miracles. So it is touching to see Paul's concern in and love for his co-worker, Epaphroditus, who had been sick and almost died (Philippians 2). The crisis of sickness really bonded him with Epaphroditus.

Sometimes people write that they are afraid to tell their kids about their cancer diagnosis. Some share very little of their battle with their kids. I certainly understand this, as cancer is hard for adults to understand. Still, I wonder if kids are more resilient than we think. They need to understand that their parents are vulnerable and even a bit scared, but that they can turn to the Lord for courage and strength. After all, kids need to be equipped to handle hard situations and how to show value to others when they are weak. Finding strength and comfort is a joint effort when we experience helplessness together.

Lord, help us to greatly cherish and value every moment with the important people in our lives.

Secondhand Pain

terri fornear

*Not that we are adequate in ourselves to consider anything as coming from ourselves,
but our adequacy is from God.*

2 Corinthians 3:5

Do you ever feel like you're not going to make it through a situation? Empty of hope and seeing no answers? That is how I feel when I watch someone I love in pain. Whether the pain is physical or emotional, I feel my own helplessness to its full extent. I do not handle these times very well. Anxiety roars and fears chase my heart into hiding. I become paralyzed.

Once again I'm beginning to take tiny baby steps through hard times. Psalm 68:28 was one of my first steps. "Summon your power, O God. Show me your strength, O God, as you have done before." Then I found a great quote from the devotional book, *Streams in the Desert*:

He becomes my strength to sit still. What a difficult accomplishment this is! If I could only do something! I feel like the mother who stands by her sick child but is powerless to heal. What a severe test. Yet to do nothing except to sit still and wait requires tremendous strength.

He becomes my strength to watch without answers. He becomes my strength to handle anxious thoughts that cloud my mind. He helps me take each thought captive to Jesus. His Life within me carries me through fears I cannot overcome on my own.

To the outside world I may look void of faith and hope. When Jesus was on the cross, they shouted, "Where is your God now? Let Him deliver you." I am tempted to feel like a failure as a Christian. The battle is in full rage. Yet this is not the time to look at myself or measure my faith. I must look away to Jesus, who was not impressive on that cross. He was considered a loser. So I go to Him for that same strength which helped Him stay on that cross.

He's giving me His heart for my beloved who is in pain. He is praying through me for deliverance of that pain and for wisdom for the next step. He is interceding through me. "I have been crucified with Christ; and it is no longer I who live, but Christ lives in me; and the life which I now live in the flesh I live by faith in the Son of God, who loved me and gave Himself up for me" (Galatians 2:20). The Lord is my strength.

Lord, live through us so that we can handle the intensity of our own battles
and to be able to help others in their battles.

Advice from a Weak One Made Strong

joe fornear

For we do not want you to be unaware, brethren, of our affliction which came to us in Asia,
that we were burdened excessively, beyond our strength, so that
we despaired even of life; indeed, we had the sentence of death within ourselves
so that we would not trust in ourselves, but in God who raises the dead.

2 Corinthians 1:8–9

Kalisha Frazier of UV Skinz interviewed Joe Fornear about his battle with cancer and his book, *My Stronghold, A Pastor's Battle with Cancer and Doubts*. UV Skinz makes clothing and other products that protect the skin from ultraviolet rays. Kalisha asked some penetrating questions.

Question: You have been down a long road—do you have any advice to those in the midst of battling cancer?

I think my best advice is to embrace your weakness. God never intended for us to handle cancer alone. When I was in the midst of the roughest times during my fight, I tried so hard to be strong. The problem was that I had become so weary; I had no natural strength left to fight. I was frustrated with myself that I couldn't rise above the pain and sadness. I kind of beat myself up, because I thought I should be stronger. It was okay for me to admit I was weak, even though I was a big, tough guy from Pittsburgh, the Steel City. One of my favorite Bible passages is 2 Corinthians 12:9 and 10, "And He has said to me, 'My grace is sufficient for you, for power is perfected in weakness.' Most gladly, therefore, I will rather boast about my weaknesses, so that the power of Christ may dwell in me."

Question: You mention that you developed a "spiteful awe of cancer" during this experience. Can you explain how it affected your outlook on beating your disease?

When I began the surgeries and treatments, I wasn't totally committed to the battle. Stage IV melanoma is a very serious disease, and it is unwise to fight it in a half-hearted way. Early on, I had a type of denial, that I was going to get through this quickly, and I didn't need to "baby" myself. After my two surgeries on the lymph nodes under my arm, I still kept pushing myself. I didn't want to miss any of my kids' (Jesse and Amy) high school basketball games. This complicated my recovery. I was running around in the rain and cold and got a staph infection which carried over to the third surgery to remove one-third of my stomach. I really didn't want to be in the battle, yet to fight effectively, I needed to surrender to the fact that I was in a real battle and I needed to get my heart and head into the fight.

Still in the end, I don't claim to have beaten the disease myself. In May 2003, my doctor told me I had days to live because melanoma had spread to both sides of my pancreas, lung, kidney, pelvis and several other sites. The doctor had basically given up on me. Only God could have stepped into turn my situation around. I look at it this way—Stage IV metastatic melanoma was way bigger than me, and I have no problem admitting that it got the best of me. But God is way bigger than any disease. If He decides to keep you around, you will stay. It took a miracle for me, and I know I am blessed to have received one.

Question: What were your feelings when you found out that you were one of the rare cases of melanoma that did not have a "primary" source of cancer and that it had spread directly to your lymph nodes?

My huge disappointment was that I was misdiagnosed by my family doctor for months. He thought I had a cyst. He has apologized for missing my diagnosis, and I have forgiven him, but he said twice during appointments about the growing lump under my arm, "Whatever it is, it's not cancer. It is too soft to be cancer." Frankly, I would have preferred to catch the disease as a skin lesion in Stage I, but God had other plans. I can see now why He allowed it. But, people should know, melanoma is never to be taken lightly and can present itself in uncommon ways, like not having a skin lesion, but having the melanoma spread directly to lymph nodes. I recommend getting your skin checked by a dermatologist once a year, and always get a second opinion on any lumps on your body.

Question: What changes have you made to your lifestyle to continue to boost your immune system?

I eat a lot better with less food overall, and a lot less sugar. I have worked less and slept more, as I have some serious workaholic tendencies. I also try not to not get worked up about life's frustrations as stress wears down our immunities. I have learned to cast my anxiety and frustration on the Lord more. This helps immensely. He is my Stronghold in hard times and in everyday life as well.

Question: How has cancer become a gift in your life?

During my battle, when someone first mentioned to me that cancer was such a gift to her, I thought that was one of the dumbest things I'd ever heard. Now though I see how the Lord has used my cancer battle in many ways. A short list:

- I have much more compassion for weakness and for suffering than ever. We launched Stronghold Ministry because of this. We help cancer patients through their battle.
- I learned so much about the Lord and grew closer to Him. I now share this knowledge of Him with everyone I can, and certainly with cancer patients and caretakers.
- I learned how fragile life is, and respect my own health more.
- I have reconnected with old friends from college and high school. They were instrumental in encouraging me and inspiring me to hang on. I also reconnected so much deeper with my seven siblings and my mother as they were a huge support to me.
- My wife Terri was such an angelic gift to me. We definitely have been changed by the whole experience, and the battle has helped our marriage. We appreciate each other more for sure.

Question: The day you found out you were cured—what was that moment like?

At first I didn't believe it. We had taken the PET scan images home immediately after the test before the radiologist had even looked at the images. We looked at them and concluded the cancer had spread even more. We misread the scans, obviously. So when the radiologist's report read that I was NED (no evidence of disease), it was kind of surreal, but eventually the news sunk in and we really celebrated. My doctor was so cautious though, and said, "Now you have nine months to live." But I proclaimed myself cured and told him all chemo would cease immediately. He talked me out of that, and I finished the remaining three rounds. I had several false alarms since 2003, when doctors said the cancer had come back. Five years is the official medical threshold when melanoma patients are considered cured. It took that long for me to feel cured. But almost every day along the way, I have thanked God for His kindness to me.

Lord, all glory goes to You for healing Joe. Use our battle to reach others for you.

ABIDING

♡

Abiding in a Besieged City

terri fornear

For this is the covenant that I will make with the house of Israel after those days, says the Lord: I will put my laws into their minds, and I will write them on their hearts. And I will be their God, and they shall be my people. And they shall not teach everyone his fellow citizen, and everyone his brother, saying, 'Know the Lord,' for all will know Me, from the least to the greatest of them.

Hebrews 8:10–11

I remember Christmas Day in 2002, when we received the news that Joe had "metastatic melanoma." I remember the tree lights, the candles in church, the neighborhood lights—and the darkness in my heart. I felt like we were the only ones in the neighborhood who couldn't seem to hang house lights.

I also remember feeling at the time that Jesus' birth didn't seem to have a lot of relevance to cancer. I was like the nation of Israel in Jeremiah's day, when God said in Jeremiah 32:33, "They turned their backs to Me and not their faces." Before the cancer hit, I'm really not sure how much God was seeing my face. I was busy doing His work, having Bible studies, decorating the church, buying gifts for those I love and dressing outwardly in the Christmas spirit. When I heard Joe had cancer, it stopped me cold. I had to meet Him face-to-face.

Like the people in Israel, we were in a besieged city, a walled-up city, with an enemy surrounding us. Yet His ultimate goal was to bless them—and bless us. Then I read Jeremiah 32:38:

> They shall be My people, and I will be their God; and I will give them one heart and one way, that they may fear Me always, for their own good and for the good of their children after them. I will make an everlasting covenant with them that I will not turn away from them, to do them good; and I will put the fear of Me in their hearts so that they will not turn away from Me. I will rejoice over them to do them good and will faithfully plant them in this land with all My heart and with all My soul.

What "land" does He plant me in? It is the land of the Life of Jesus. He does something miraculous in the person that receives His gift of Jesus into their heart. He transforms that heart. He has given us a new covenant which provides a new heart which follows Him. This heart can look Him straight in His face with no hint of condemnation, and is able to receive His rejoicing over us. It is a heart that makes us His child and heir to all that the Father has for us.

One of His greatest gifts is boldness to come into His throne room, approach Him face to face and ask whatever we wish. Jesus said in John 15:7, "If you abide in Me, and My words abide in you, ask whatever you wish, and it will be done for you." Do we believe our wishes could be His? Do we know that He has given us His heart and He will lead this heart into His good places with Him?

Jesus' birth has much relevance to fighting cancer and *everything* we face.

Lord, fill us with appreciation for the birth of Your Son who gave us a brand new relationship with You in which we know Your heart.

Abiding in the valley

terri fornear

Thus says the Lord, "Because the Syrians have said, 'The Lord is a god of the hills but he is not a god of the valleys,' therefore I will give all this great multitude into your hand and you shall know that I am the Lord."

1 Kings 20:28

Why do I think I am close to God only when I see His blessing? Is He with me only when my children are flourishing with success and happiness, when everyone is healthy, when friends pursue the friendship, when money is no object, when my hair looks great? Then I hear that "Syrian" voice, "Your God is only a god of the hills and mountain tops."

The valleys feel lonely, dark and fearful. I am truly lost and confused when evil and trials touch my life. My eyes are focused on life, not His life, but my life. Why do I get so distracted with the good when I have the best?

He opens my eyes—down there—in the valley. I see the real war He is fighting this side of eternity. This is a war which He has been preparing an army to fight, equipping them in invisible realms. He fits them with the only weapon that can break through to truth and to Him—His Son's Life.

His Son is released inside of the weak, the humble and the empty, so He can show Himself to the world He died to love. "To whom God willed to make known what is the riches of the glory of this mystery among the Gentiles, which is Christ in you, the hope of glory" (Colossians 1:27).

In the valley, where we feel invisible, He is making Himself visible.

Lord, show us that You are indeed the God of the valleys as well as the mountains.

Abiding While I Wait
In Unanswered Prayer

terri fornear

*Simon Peter then, having a sword, drew it and struck the high priest's slave, and cut off his right ear;
and the slave's name was Malchus. So Jesus said to Peter, "Put the sword into the sheath;
the cup which the Father has given Me, shall I not drink it? Or do you think that I cannot appeal
to My Father, and He will at once put at My disposal more than twelve legions of angels?"*

Matthew 26:52-53

Sometimes I feel like God is a million miles away. As a caretaker, I watch the pain of the one I love—physical pain, pain from rejection and failure, and pain as dreams crumble. The Lord doesn't seem to answer what I think is an urgent plea. I do not *feel* the love that everyone claims God has and is. I'm helpless to fix. Watching without being able to change anything brings me to the end of my resources faster than anything.

Jesus then shows me the road He walked that day He went to the cross. He had perfect surrender and perfect rest. He didn't need Peter's sword or Peter's help. He knew He had a Father that could unleash a legion of protective angels to deliver Him. And His Father was not planning to deliver Him at that moment. He did not fight. He kept walking toward the cup He was asked to drink.

Sometimes when my cup is full of watching others hurt, I want to pull out my sword and make a way of clarity and smoothness for them. He helps me put that sword away as I abide in *His* ability to trust the Father when I can't. He reminds me that God's love is full of purpose. The cup of pain I see others drink will lead to the same resurrected life which Jesus experienced.

*Lord, it is so hard to stand by helplessly and watch people we love suffer,
but though You could stop their pain in a second, You plan great blessings for the suffering.*

Abiding In His Reconciliation

terri fornear

But God demonstrates His own love for us in this: While we were still sinners, Christ died for us.
For if, when we were God's enemies, we were reconciled to him through the death of his Son,
how much more, having been reconciled, shall we be saved through his life.

Romans 5:8 &10

Why do I continually think I have to make myself worthy for God to love? I do it in so many ways. I try to make all of my relationships peaceful and right. I try to think and do all of the right things. I try to be a good wife, mother and friend. All this trying, yet I always seem to come up short in someone's eyes. I pray, read my Bible, care and still come up short.

Then I catch a glimpse of Jesus' walk to the cross. Lining the road were people who misunderstood Him. They spat on Him, mocked Him and called Him a liar. He went to the cross for His enemies. His enemies were all those who did not believe in Him—his persecutors, those who pounded the nails into His hands, even His own fearful disciples. In a way, I was also on that road of unbelief. I basically call Him a liar when I do not believe His love which He gave that day. He went to the cross when I was still a sinner, and still His enemy. He reconciled me to Himself—not because I loved Him and saw who He was. He loved me first (1 John 4:19). He reconciled me, because He really is love. So if He did that when I was His enemy, as He says in the passages in Romans 5, how much more will He save my life through His life?

He came to save the sick, the weak and the sinner who disbelieves. He gave His heart and life to me when He walked to that cross. My inability to perform just helps me take what He has freely given—without all of the trying! "Therefore I will boast all the more gladly of my weaknesses, so that the power of Christ may rest upon me. … For when I am weak, then I am strong" (2 Corinthians 12:9, 10).

♡

Lord, when people don't reconcile with me,
help me remember that it was You who first reconciled with me.

Abiding in His Protection
terri fornear

For by their own sword they did not possess the land, and their own arm did not save them, but Your right hand and Your arm and the light of Your presence, for You favored them. You are my King, O God; Command victories for Jacob. Through You we will push back our adversaries. Through Your name we will trample down those who rise up against us. For I will not trust in my bow, nor will my sword save me. But You have saved us from our adversaries, and You have put to shame those who hate us. In God we have boasted all day long, and we will give thanks to Your name.

Psalm 44:3-8

Some days just seem evil. There are days when the messages in my head are so negative. I can't seem to fight them. I think that is what Paul meant by "the day of evil" (Ephesians 6:13). These are days of inadequacies and confusion. Days when I realize I am vulnerable, weak and losing my grip and overwhelmed.

He never said I had to fight my own battles. In fact, He said that if I did, I would lose. I cannot trust in my "bow," which means my weapons to try to win the battle. My schemes, ideas, medicines, doctors, friends and family all fall short in one way or another. In Him alone do I boast. My cry to Him brings victory. He comes through as I hide myself in His Word. He is my refuge and protection.

You come to me, Lord, with "Your right arm." (This we now know is the work of Jesus who is sitting at Your right side saying, "I have already won this victory—let's give it to her now.")

You come with "the light of Your presence." (Jesus, the light of this world, cannot be snuffed out. He overcomes the darkness.)

You come with Your "favor." (Because of Jesus' life in me, I am favored forever.)

♡

Lord, I want to snuggle up in Your arms with Your Son, and watch as You show Your glory today.

Abiding In Persevering Faith

terri fornear

If you abide in Me, and My words abide in you, ask whatever you wish, and it will be done for you.

John 15:7

These are words that I heard loud and clear, and it was done for me. My wish for Joe's healing was granted! So why now do I doubt the small stuff? My heart grieves because of my "little faith" after such a big answer.

Why do I fear getting headaches?

Why do I fear failing in a new job?

Why do I struggle with relationships?

Why do I think calamity is around every corner?

If I were God I would hang me out to dry—on a very windy day!

But He's not like that with His amazing grace and amazing voice. Once more I hear, "Terri, let Me be your dwelling place." He declares in the Psalms that He has been our dwelling place for all generations, but am I living in it? The Israelites had His Presence, but still wandered in the wilderness. They found no city and they were hungry and their souls fainted. The truth is our souls are made for God. He is our home and we will never find rest outside of Him.

The Lord is my Rock,
My Fortress,
My Deliverer.

What safer abiding place is there? Oh, my soul, believe and rest.

♡

Lord, You've done such great things in our lives, help us to remember You never leave us.

God, Can You Really Relate?

joe fornear

For we do not have a high priest who cannot sympathize with our weaknesses,
but One who has been tempted in all things as we are, yet without sin.

Hebrews 4:15

I think we can let our imaginations run with this verse. When Jesus the carpenter smacked his thumb with a hammer, I'm sure, like us, He was tempted to cuss at the top of His lungs. At the end of Jesus' work days, He knew what it is like to be tired, even totally exhausted. He has felt the grouchiness that hunger brings. When the town beauty queen walked by and all the carpenters began whistling and commenting, I'm sure He was tempted to stare at her in inappropriate ways. As this verse in Hebrews sates, He was certainly tempted in *all* ways.

Jesus was such an amazingly loving person, so surely everyone loved Him, right? No, and that is sad. He seemed to accumulate more and more enemies. He was tempted to compromise to cause people to like Him. He didn't budge and as a result, the Bible says, "He was despised and forsaken of men, a man of sorrows and acquainted with grief. And like one from whom men hide their face He was despised, and we did not esteem Him" (Isaiah 53:3). He knows how it feels to be left out, forgotten, even deliberately ostracized. He absorbed false accusations and even forgave His betrayers. He graciously endured being framed in court and took the ultimate fall of a death penalty—all for us.

He endured the full range of human experience and all without error. One might think His success as a human rendered Him intolerant of our bumbling ways, but this is not the case at all! He knows the journey is tough for us, as it was tough for Him. The next verse in Hebrews 4:16 reveals the depth of His empathy. "Therefore let us draw near with confidence to the throne of grace, so that we may receive mercy and find grace to help in time of need." There is no hint of condemnation, just an open invitation to the undeserving to draw near for grace and mercy.

He understands that we struggle, and He knows exactly why, and yet He is still so willing to help!

Lord, we know You can relate,
so we ask You to provide Your experienced help in getting us through our battles.

Priming the Pump: How to Keep Living Waters Flowing

joe fornear

If anyone is thirsty, let him come to Me and drink. He who believes in Me, as the Scripture said, "From his innermost being will flow rivers of living water."

John 7:37-38

In this verse, Jesus diagnosed the spiritual condition of the religious at one of the Jewish feasts. There was an epidemic of spiritual dehydration and so He offered to quench their thirst with "living water." Sadly, religion can be reduced to man's vain attempts to gain God's love and approval. When we pursue God's love or human love in this manner, we dry up.

Ironically, Jesus offered this same living water to a woman in Samaria who had been searching for approval and love from men. Jesus perceived that she was determined to switch partners until she found love, so He offered her a truly satisfying *internal* love.

People are not so different after all. Both the religious and the promiscuous yearn for acceptance, affirmation and satisfaction. Our methods and means may vary, but our goals are the same. As a result, we all experience the same spiritual dryness. The remedy for our thirst is the same as well. It is the living water which only Jesus provides.

Jesus steers us to the source of that water, the person of the Holy Spirit. He has been placed inside of everyone who believes in Christ as their personal Savior. This is what it means to be born again; the Holy Spirit makes a person come alive to God after being dead in sin. This living water is available and ready to flow in and out of us, but it needs to be tapped.

So how do we prime the pump?

Drop our bucket into the right well. If we drink from the world's wells of sin, escape and amusement, it is no wonder we remain thirsty. God told Jonah, "Those who cling to worthless idols, forfeit the grace that could be theirs" (Jonah 2:8). Don't be determined to find love in all the wrong places.

Don't push away the hand that serves the drink. If we are angry and disillusioned with God, we don't experience His joy or the flow of His Spirit. We may be angry, as the Proverb says, because we have placed our hope in some earthly, temporal goal, which is a recipe for hopelessness. "Hope deferred makes the heart sick" (Proverbs 13:12). Though our bodies are physically sick, our hearts can be spiritually healthy. Don't drift away from the One who can give you internal health.

Throughout the Scriptures, God allows His children to suffer. Yet out of that suffering He works all things to our ultimate good and to His glory. "And we know that God causes all things to work together for good to those who love God, to those who are called according to His purpose" (Romans 8:28). Tragedies and setbacks can either make us bitter or better. If we take God at His word, we will trust He will work something good out of heart-breaking hardships.

Slow down and drink up. Picture a marathon runner who wishes to grab a cup of water during a race. He must slow down enough to complete a clean hand off. If he refuses to slow down, he will continue to knock cups to the ground or spill the water out of the cups. The result is that he stays thirsty. Many people are like this runner. Some are running toward something, while others are running away from something. Many fear slowing down as their inner drive takes over common sense. Psalm 46:10, "Cease striving and know that I am God." Give Him a chance to be God in your life.

God is not impressed with how much we do. He can accomplish far more *through* us than we can accomplish *for* Him. So slow down and take daily drinks from God's deep well of satisfying spiritual water. He is the ultimate source of love, acceptance and satisfaction. Then we will have something to give to others and will not feel so dry and drained. We have to get under the spout where His glory comes out!

Lord, help us slow down and drink deeply from the well of the Holy Spirit whom You have placed inside of us.

SUPPORT
of
PEOPLE

Holding Up the Hurting
joe fornear

*So it came about when Moses held his hand up, that Israel prevailed,
and when he let his hand down, Amalek prevailed. But Moses' hands were heavy …
and Aaron and Hur supported his hands, one on one side and one on the other.
Thus his hands were steady until the sun set. So Joshua overwhelmed Amalek.*

Exodus 17:11-13

This 3500-year-old account of the battle at Rephidim is so applicable today. It reveals a fascinating interplay between prayer, God's intervention and supporting each other in our individual battles. We are all like Moses, fighting fierce battles. Whether we are fighting cancer or working through life's many trials, in some ways we all must fight alone. Yet this passage teaches our prayers and faith for each other can influence unseen enemy forces.

We believe the Lord has called Stronghold Ministry to be like Aaron and Hur. We come alongside cancer warriors to help hold up their hands in battle. We are a tool in God's hand to lighten many loads. We operate in spiritual realms, in arenas of the mind, in deep recesses of the cancer patient's heart where even their closest friends may not go. Many call or write us right before their surgery or treatments to seek our prayers and encouragement. Many let down their guards and express critical concerns.

Yet Stronghold Ministry needs help to hold up the weary arms of hurting people. Could you hold us up in prayer? Could you commit to pray for our patients? Also, please pray for our ministry, that we would be bold and sensitive with God's Word.

Let us know of your battles, too. We want to hold up your arms for victory.

♡

Lord, help us hold up in prayer those who are hurting in their battles with unseen enemies.

Caretakers: Not Your Average Joes

joe fornear

Joseph, son of David, do not be afraid to take Mary as your wife;
for the Child who has been conceived in her is of the Holy Spirit. She will bear a Son;
and you shall call His name Jesus, for He will save His people from their sins.

Matthew 1:20-21

Multitudes of sermons and devotionals revolve around Mary, wise men and shepherds, but have you heard many sermons about Joseph? Often the animals surrounding Jesus' birth are given more consideration than Joseph. So why is Jesus' earthly father overlooked despite his substantial contribution to the events of the birth of the Son of God?

Perhaps Joseph is taken for granted because he did what was expected. He simply took good care of Mary and Jesus. Yet he was a very effective caretaker. From a human perspective, He was called to fight for the very life of his young son. He literally "saved" the Savior's life. The evil King Herod was exceedingly threatened by news of a Messiah King's birth. He determined to snuff out this rival at an early age by killing all of the young boys. Warned by an angel in a dream, Joseph picked up his young family and fled to Egypt until Herod died. Certainly God held Jesus and Joseph in His sovereign grip. Still, what a great weight Joseph must have carried!

In honor of Joseph, the unsung hero, we want to recognize and encourage all of the caretakers of our cancer patients. Their physical, emotional and spiritual needs are often overshadowed by the intensity of the patient's fight. Yet what great weights they often carry, while feeling so responsible and yet so helpless all at the same time!

Many caretakers, like my wife Terri, fight tirelessly for their patient. Several times during my battle with Stage IV metastatic melanoma, I had no strength or will to press on. Yet God used Terri to help carry me through.

Now it is not the responsibility of caretakers to "save" their loved ones. Those decisions are made in God's sovereign plans. Ultimately, God chose to spare me, yet I have profound admiration for so many who have not had the same outcome as Terri and I. Their pain and grief far surpasses ours, and they have handled their profound losses with amazing grace and dignity.

Please pray for the caretakers of the world, and encourage the ones you know. If you feel led, contact a caretaker and tell them you admire them. They might be doing what is expected, but so many have performed an impossible task so well!

Lord, we ask You to touch the caretakers with Your supernatural peace, strength, comfort and love.
Let them know their tender care does not escape Your notice.

How to Help Cancer Patients and Caretakers

joe fornear

I was sick and you visited Me.

Matthew 25:36

Jesus cares about the sick. He gives us guidance on how to help them in many passages in Scripture. The following are some ideas on how to help:

Really pray. I'll admit it; sometimes I have told someone, "I am praying," but did not follow through. We should not just say that we will pray. Pray with the sick, and also pray for them as often as you think of them. If it made no difference, I can't imagine the Lord telling us to "pray without ceasing" (1 Thessalonians 5:17)!

Don't underestimate the value of your presence. Fight the urge to be profound, just "being there" is a huge statement of compassion and care. Be careful of spouting true, but ill-timed clichés. While it's true that God works all things out for the good, someone might be better off with a hug or simply praying together.

Listen well. Every person is different; every situation is different. Let people approach their battle in their way. "Counsel in the heart of man is like deep water; but a man of understanding will draw it out" (Proverbs 20:5). If you've never had cancer, do not say, "I know how you feel." Say instead, "I can only imagine how you feel."

Let the patient/caretaker take the emotional lead. "Rejoice with those who rejoice, and weep with those who weep" (Romans 12:15). Allow people to have negative feelings. Job, David, Gideon and even Jesus were upset and distressed. "My God, my God, why have you forsaken me?"

Do not judge. Don't be like Job's friends; lose all of those judgmental thoughts about the cause of another's cancer. If God gave everyone cancer in exchange for their sin, we would all have it and never be rid of it!

Be careful with advice. The longer I operate in this world of cancer, the more respect I have for the professionals. They're not perfect, but they know a lot more than I do. If I make a medical suggestion, I always try to add, "But check with your doctor on this." A treatment that worked for one person may not work for another. And, please don't forward letters from experts and hospitals who actually deny composing them, that some supplement, or asparagus, or oxygen has been proven to cure cancer. Some remedies might help a patient fight cancer, but there is yet to be a simple cure that "they" don't want us to know. Think about it for a moment—if a legitimate cure existed, wouldn't everyone know by now?

Give practically. Food and money almost always help. Most cancer patients are usually short on money because of the costs of battling cancer, reduced work hours, traveling for treatment, insurance co-pays and deductibles and extra supplements or nutritional programs. Every bit of financial help means so much.

Be hopeful. Hope is always good, so be positive. A Christian doctor once hopelessly said to me, "You're getting people's hopes up—you should just be preparing them to die," but I'd rather die with hope, than live with no hope. Yet don't be extreme in conveying hope. I did not feel hopeful when people told me, "You're going to beat this." It was as if they were saying I had the power to get rid of cancer, but I quickly learned I could not just will it away. Only the Lord determines the number of our days. So instead tell them, "With God's help, and the doctor's help and our help, you're going to beat this."

Lord, make us like You, sensitive and compassionate, so that we can truly help the hurting and sick.

Lessons from Geese

joe fornear

Two are better than one because they have a good return for their labor. For if either of them falls, the one will lift up his companion. But woe to the one who falls when there is not another to lift him up. Furthermore, if two lie down together they keep warm, but how can one be warm alone? And if one can overpower him who is alone, two can resist him. A cord of three strands is not quickly torn apart.

Ecclesiastes 4:9–12

Most folks observe geese only when a flock soars overhead. Yet insights from these fascinating birds can teach us powerful lessons about life. First, do you know why one side of their V-shaped flight formations are often longer than the other? Well, because there are more birds on that side! But seriously, take a "gander" at these amazing facts and lessons from the goose:

Fact 1: As each goose flaps its wings it creates "lift" for the other birds that follow. By flying in V formation, the whole flock adds 71 percent greater flying range than if each bird flew alone. When a goose falls out of formation, it feels the drag and resistance of flying alone. It quickly moves back into formation to take advantage of the lifting power of the bird immediately in front of it.

Lesson: It is no surprise that God asks us to "fly" together. 1 Thessalonians 5:14 says, "We urge you, brethren, admonish the unruly, encourage the fainthearted, help the weak, be patient with everyone."

Fact 2: When the lead goose tires, it rotates back into the formation and another goose flies to the point position.

Lesson: No one person has the strength or ability to be the point person in all the different areas of life. We all have to step up and play some part in making others strong. We are interdependent on each other's skills, capabilities and unique arrangements of gifts, talents and resources.

Fact 3: The geese flying in formation "honk" to encourage those in front to keep up their speed.

Lesson: We need to make sure our "honking" is encouraging. In groups where there is much encouragement, the production is much greater. Think of the home field advantage in sports. Is our goal to find what is good in each other or to pinpoint each other's faults?

Fact 4: When a goose gets sick or wounded, two geese drop out of formation and follow it to the ground to help and protect it. They stay with the sick bird until it is able to fly again. Then they launch out with another formation or catch up with their original flock.

Lesson: We all struggle at some point in our lives, and we all need each other's help. Yet the reaction of some people to others' troubles is, "Glad it's them and not me." But Paul says in 1 Corinthians 12:26, "If one member suffers, all the members suffer with it." If you stub your big toe, your whole body knows it, doesn't it? Are you tuned in to help alleviate the pain of others? Help others as you would have them help you. Let's form a "V."

Lord, these birds which You have designed,
teach us amazing lessons about Your warmth and compassion for the hurting.

What Not To Say to a Cancer Patient

joe fornear

Some boast in chariots and some in horses, but we will boast in the name of the LORD, our God.

Psalm 20:7

Biblical authors often spoke out about trusting in horses and chariots rather than depending on the Lord to win battles. People in every time period have displayed this tendency to place all of our trust in their own weapons and talents. In our cancer battles, we should certainly find and utilize the best weapons we possibly can, but ultimately our success is in the Lord's hands.

This is why I recommend *not* saying this common encouragement to a cancer patient: "You're going to beat this," especially with late-stage warriors. It is a bold claim which seems to exude optimism and instill inspiration. So how could it possibly be an unwise statement? Unfortunately, it places the burden of ultimate victory squarely on the patient. Most patients desperately want to get well. They are probably doing more than you realize to recover, but having the responsibility to get better can be overwhelming. Positive thinking will not remove all of their cancer cells.

Please keep this in mind, no matter how tough your patient appears, most are weaker than they claim. How do I know this? They tell me so in private that few people grasp what they are really going through. I also felt that way myself during my own battle. There is tremendous pressure on patients to remain positive so that their caretakers and network do not become fearful and depressed.

Lance Armstrong seems to be the epitome of the triumph of the human spirit. I have great admiration for the tenacity he brought to his cancer fight and his accomplishments afterwards as well. Yet "living strong" has its limits. Consider what his longtime coach and confidante, Chris Carmichael, said in a newspaper interview:

> People believe that Lance is a tough guy: He beat cancer, he willed it away. They think he left this Earth and is invincible. That's far from the truth. He

has the same mortality as anyone else. He dealt with cancer the same way as anyone else. I saw him scared and fearful, with all the human emotions associated with that intense experience (*USA TODAY*, May 22, 2002).

Doctors and modern medicine have come a long way and the Lord uses doctors to save lives on a daily basis. Yet our trust should not be exclusively placed in doctors or treatments. When King Asa was sick, he made the mistake of not seeking the Lord at all. He relied entirely on the doctors. "In the thirty-ninth year of his reign, Asa became diseased in his feet. His disease was severe, yet even in his disease he did not seek the LORD, but the physicians (2 Chronicles 16:12).

To really love someone in the midst of crisis we should follow Paul's advice and "Weep with those who weep" (Romans 12:15). And, "To the weak I became weak, that I might win the weak" (1 Corinthians 9:22). We may want to lift strugglers out of weakness with just a turn of a phrase, but that rarely works.

People need to feel unconditionally accepted, understood and supported, especially in a crisis. They need to look to the Lord more than to the doctors or themselves. If they have permission to be weak around you, ironically, they will be able to draw strength from you and the Lord. By all means, be positive and full of hope. I think it's best to say, "With the doctor's help, and your friends and family's help, and especially the Lord's help, we will beat this."

Lord, our trust is in You alone, for what is impossible with man is possible with You.

FORGIVENESS

♡

Pardon Me!: God's Forgiveness

joe fornear

*When the natives saw the creature hanging from his hand, they began saying to one another,
"Undoubtedly this man is a murderer, and though he has been saved from the sea,
justice has not allowed him to live."*

Acts 28:4

Paul had survived a fierce storm and was shipwrecked on an island. The natives of the island welcomed his crew, but when they saw him get bit by a snake, they drew very judgmental conclusions that were eventually proven false. They reasoned that Paul must have done something deserving death and punishment, as justice had apparently caught up with him—or so they thought.

Not much has changed since Paul's day as some people today believe cancer is a punishment from God. Some cancer patients may wonder if they are being punished by God. This is a distressing issue for many who find themselves in this fiery trial. After all, who can look back on their lives and declare themselves sin-free? If you need a hint: only the helplessly self-righteous.

But this is not how God deals with those who have received His Son and our Savior, Jesus Christ! This is the reason Christ came to earth: to *take away* our punishment so that we could walk away free men and women! Isaiah 53:5–6 puts it like this:

> But He was pierced through for our transgressions; He was crushed for our iniquities. The chastening for our well-being fell upon Him, and by His scourging we are healed. All of us like sheep have gone astray, each of us has turned to his own way, but the Lord has caused the iniquity of us all to fall on Him.

In the American justice system, presidents can "pardon" those accused of crimes. They can release criminals from prison, and even clear their records, as if they had never done anything wrong. This is what God does for us in Christ. He officially and forever pardons us. What president pardons someone and then punishes them for the offense anyway? This would not be pardon at all.

Consider two additional promises of His mercy and forgiveness:

- I will cleanse them from all their iniquity by which they have sinned against Me, and I will pardon all their iniquities by which they have sinned against Me and by which they have transgressed against Me (Jeremiah 33:8).
- I, even I, am the one who wipes out your transgressions for My own sake, and I will not remember your sins (Isaiah 43:25).

The second verse says that He doesn't even remember our sins, so why would He still punish us for them? True, if God wanted to, He could certainly *recall* our sins, but He chooses to forget about them. Clearly, He is promising that He won't ever punish us for them. These promises apply to all of our sins: past, present and future. Could it be any other way? Certainly we will all sin in the future. Yet those sins are covered by His forgiveness as well!

Some might think such mercy is an incentive to sin, but why would anyone deliberately disobey a God with such amazing love for us?

Thank You, oh merciful Lord, for Your incredible plan to pardon my sin!

Resolving the Past

joe fornear

Search me, O God, and know my heart; Try me and know my anxious thoughts.

Psalms 139:23

Let's be real, we all accumulate baggage on life's journeys. We are loaded down with shortcomings, regrets and sins. So how do we resolve these issues so that we can live free in the here and now? How do we rid ourselves of guilt?

Simply confess your sins. Who hasn't mistreated, neglected or spoken unkindly about another? Who hasn't disobeyed God's will in some area? I've sinned in countless ways—coveting, lying, stealing and cheating—just to name a few areas. How about you?

The guilt of our sins can plague us, especially when we're sick. Yet there is relief—we can take on the righteousness of Another. The great apostle Paul sought to be righteous, but surprisingly, he did not seek righteousness by doing good deeds. "Not having a righteousness of my own derived from the Law, but that which is through faith in Christ, the righteousness which comes from God on the basis of faith" (Philippians 3:9).

John tells us *how* to receive Christ's righteousness, by simply admitting and confessing our sins, and by faith receiving the forgiveness and righteousness of Jesus Christ, our Advocate.

If we confess our sins, He is faithful and righteous to forgive us our sins and to cleanse us from all unrighteousness (I John 1:9).

And if anyone sins, we have an Advocate with the Father, Jesus Christ the righteous. And He Himself is the propitiation for our sins (1 John 2:1–2).

Relinquish your regrets. We may be confident of God's forgiveness, but have we forgiven ourselves? We've all blown it; we've all done foolish things, but punishing ourselves accomplishes nothing. Jeremiah 31:34 says about His forgiveness, "For I will forgive their iniquity and their sin I will remember no more." We should forgive and forget our sins as well! "But one thing I do: forgetting what lies behind and reaching forward to what lies ahead" (Philippians 3:13). Don't hold yourself to a higher standard than God's—that's just pride.

Cut yourself slack for your shortcomings. We've all been letdown by others, but sometimes we are letdown most by ourselves! After doctors told me I had days to live in 2003, I slipped down into a pit of disappointment. I was grieved that I had not accomplished more in my 44 years. I had big goals and had fallen well-short. While goals are crucial, chastising oneself for missing them is not healthy. The root of this disappointment in myself was prideful perfectionism. Paul addresses this tendency as well in Philippians 3:12–14:

> Not that I have already obtained it or have already become perfect, but I press on so that I may lay hold of that for which also I was laid hold of by Christ Jesus. Brethren, I do not regard myself as having laid hold of it yet; but one thing I do: forgetting what lies behind and reaching forward to what lies ahead, I press on toward the goal for the prize of the upward call of God in Christ Jesus." I just need to be faithful to the goals of Jesus Christ.

Your past, my past—there is no good reason to dwell there. We should learn from the past; resolve it God's way; and then forget about it. How liberating!

Lord, help us stand in Your forgiveness and resolve the issues of our past in Your way!

To Forgive Or Not to Forgive: Forgiving Others

joe fornear

And forgive us our sins, for we ourselves also forgive everyone who is indebted to us.

Luke 11:4

If I could venture one essential requirement for people fighting cancer, it would be this: forgive those who hurt you. If your battle is anything like mine was, there are many opportunities to forgive. Sometimes people say and do insensitive things when they try to help. Some have no clue what you are going through, yet claim that they do. Some try to relate to you by telling you they know someone who just died of the same cancer. Well, thank you for sharing that! A close friend may simply avoid you.

Then there are the human errors in your medical care. My primary doctor dropped the ball several times. Twice he said during appointments about the growing lump in my armpit, "Whatever it is, it isn't cancer. It's too soft to be cancer. It's just a cyst." Later, I was assured by his receptionist that the results of a critical sonogram test confirmed that I merely had a cyst. I even explained what the technician told me during the test, "These are lymph nodes! This is not a cyst!" I didn't find out the correct results until a month later. I had taken my sick daughter to him and mentioned the cyst was still growing. When I asked again about the test results, he located the report and read it for ostensibly the first time. From a human standpoint, my doctor's compounding of errors almost cost my life. Eventually he asked forgiveness for his mistakes, but he denied any wrong doing at first. For my own well-being, I realized I needed to unilaterally forgive him, whether he apologized or not.

So I have a choice, to hold things against those who have hurt me, or let it go. The following are our motivations to forgive:

Imitate Christ in being forgiving. We can look to Jesus Christ Himself. He set the tone for forgiveness for all time as He hung on the cross and said,

"Forgive them, Father, for they do not know what they are doing" (Luke 23:24). If He could forgive those who unjustly crucified Him on that humiliating cross, then we can forgive anyone—for anything!

Forgive because we've been forgiven. Since Jesus forgave us, it is only fitting that we in turn forgive others. "Be kind to one another, tender-hearted, forgiving each other, just as God in Christ also has forgiven you" (Ephesians 4:32).

Forgive because we've been forgiven so much more by God! In Matthew 18:23–35, Jesus told a lengthy parable about a guy who was forgiven an outlandish amount of money (billions of dollars), but did not extend that forgiveness to someone who owed him a fraction of that amount (merely thousands of dollars). The man wickedly demanded payment of the tiny sum. It's humbling to realize how indebted we are to Christ for forgiving such a multitude of sins. How could we fail to extend less costly forgiveness to others?

We hurt ourselves when we don't forgive. Some of us might be more inspired to forgive if we realize the consequences for holding grudges. The Bible says we hurt ourselves when we don't forgive. Notice in this verse that it is not wrong to be angry, but allowing anger to linger creates a major problem. "Be angry, and yet do not sin; do not let the sun go down on your anger, and do not give the devil an opportunity" (Ephesians 3:26–27). It does not matter what someone has done to you, let it go. The devil will try to persuade you to make an exception for some especially grievous sin committed against you. He wants to secure a foothold of bitterness in your life and bitterness is worse than cancer.

We make our pain or losses greater than God. Once when I was having a hard time forgiving someone, the Lord showed me I was considering my pain and loss to be greater than His ability to heal and restore. What wound could He not heal? What loss can He not repay tenfold? When He framed the issue in that way, it was easy for me to forgive. "The LORD is for me; I will not fear; what can man do to me?" (Psalms 118:6).

We've been insensitive ourselves. Honestly, I have said and done some very insensitive things to those who are suffering. I have avoided and neglected good friends when they needed me. So who am I to cast any stones?

Lord, grant us the grace to be merciful to others, just as You have been to us in Christ.

If God Punished All Sin with Sickness, Wouldn't You Live in a Hospital? (I Would)

joe fornear

The spirit of a man can endure his sickness, But as for a broken spirit who can bear it?
Proverbs 18:14

Once someone wrote to tell me some doctors and a pastor were researching the connection between cancer and bitterness. The "evidence" presented was that if a cancer patient was bitter toward a family member, they had cancer in a certain area of the body which the commenter specifically designated. If their bitterness was against a friend or co-worker, the cancer showed up in another specific area of the body.

Normally I would write off such quackery and cruelty, but I have encountered this erroneous thinking quite often, so I am compelled to address it here. I'll stick with God's "research," as it's conveniently packaged in the Bible.

What would we do without the powerful and freeing book of Galatians? Paul wrote to the Galatian church several years after he had started the church. I once assumed Paul had first traveled to the area to plant a church, but he actually went there for treatment for a serious eye condition.

> But you know that it was because of a bodily illness that I preached the gospel to you the first time; and that which was a trial to you in my bodily condition you did not despise or loathe, but you received me as an angel of God, as Christ Jesus Himself. Where then is that sense of blessing you had? For I bear you witness that, if possible, you would have plucked out your eyes and given them to me (Galatians 4:13–15).

Fortunately for the Galatians, they did not assume Paul's illness was a punishment for sin. Had they judged and resisted him, they would have missed their opportunity to embrace Paul's message of the grace and love of Jesus Christ!

I am a huge proponent of letting go of bitterness and turning from secret sin. We should always examine our lives and deal with sin, whether we're sick or healthy. But we should refrain from linking people's sickness to their sin. God has clearly demonstrated that He can use sickness to forge relationships and initiate many other higher purposes! So leave the judgments to Him. If God's policy was to punish all sin with sickness, wouldn't we all live in a hospital!

Lord, teach us to extend Your grace to people and not our own judgments.

FOCUS

♡

Focus

terri fornear

*The Lord GOD is my strength, and He has made my feet like hinds' feet,
and makes me walk on my high places.*

Habakkuk 3:19

You have spoken,
You have bent down and lifted me up on your shoulders.
Close to your lips.
Close to my ear.
You whisper.
"See," as you point to the end of the journey,
"Waaaay up there.

"Past the miles of hills, valleys, weeds and rivers—
a home, waiting for you.
A place where My Father—
your Father, waits for *you*."

I get distracted on the journey.
The worries, the hurts, the fears, the obstacles.
They become larger than the destiny.

I try to make this place my home.
Cozy, secure, self-protected from the elements.
Never works. Never happens.
Until you bend down and lift me up on Your shoulders,
To hear Your voice and feel Your presence.

You're my home away from home.
You are my transportation to the high places.
To My Father's Place.
My real home.
My Destination.

♡

Lord, only You can make my feet like hinds' feet—that I might reach my highest places.

The Lily of the Valley

terri fornear

I will be like the dew to Israel; He will blossom like the lily.

Hosea 14:5

During Joe's chemo treatments, I remember asking the nurses, "Has this chemo worked for others?" They would answer, "Take it a day at a time." Or, "Just enjoy every day that you're together." And, "We are all dying." Somehow at the time, those words weren't very comforting.

How do I focus each day when my life is filled with sickness and fear of losing him? Living with his pain and thinking of him as dying rattled my world. I often felt guilty thinking of myself. After all, I wasn't the one who was "suffering."

Jesus is so kind and gracious. He allowed me to ask the hard questions. He let me struggle with those true, but pat answers. He allowed me to hurt and be myself without having to pretend to be okay.

He was waiting for me to see my helplessness, because He is "the God of the valleys." My valley was surrounded by mountains of cancer which seemed immovable. They cast shadows of death. Shadows that seemed like prison walls — with no way out. Doctors told me there was less than a six percent chance of getting out. But in Hosea 14:5, Jesus Christ is likened to a lily that springs up in dark valleys with shadows of death. "The Lily of the Valley" springs up wherever He pleases.

Jesus was to me a beautiful flower. He was tall, strong and bright white. How did He get there? He was there in the valley all along. He whispered in my ear as if He had a secret. *"This Lily is in you! I am the Lily. I am the way out of the valley. I sprung up in you long ago when you first believed. Look to Me."* Jesus is the Mystery that brings Life in helpless places. I looked to Him, learned to behold Him and hope started rising in my spirit.

How this works I can't really say, but I know that the Lily, Jesus, pulls me through to triumph in the valley. Many years later, this Lily is still in me. Now I "behold" Him as I walk through new valleys. In the midst of your valleys, behold the beauty of the Lord. ♡

Lord, when we're in these desert places, spring up in our hearts with a fresh revelation of Your beauty.

Walk On!

joe fornear

And Peter got out of the boat, and walked on the water and came toward Jesus. But seeing the wind, he became frightened, and beginning to sink, he cried out, "Lord, save me!" Immediately Jesus stretched out His hand and took hold of him, and said to him, "You of little faith, why did you doubt?

Matthew 14:29-31

When you're fighting cancer, is it possible to always keep your head above water? Is it possible to be free of fear's tentacles? Just as Peter literally walked on water, this passage in Matthew 14 implies we can rise above the storms of our lives. But how?

This account is a picture of walking with Jesus through the storms of our lives. Peter was literally walking on the top of the water! He was rising above the situation—as long as He focused on Jesus. He was buoyed by His Master's confidence and serenity. As soon as he focused on the storm, he began slipping down into the deep. So the key lesson here is to focus—not on our capabilities, problems or human prognoses—but on Jesus' powers and abilities.

At their root, fears are lies about God. We should therefore face fears head on. We should let their error surface, so we can smack them down. One by one they'll lose their grip as every angle of their deceptions are held up to the light of God's love and power. Romans 8:35 and 37 encourages us, "Who will separate us from the love of Christ? Will tribulation, or distress, or persecution, or famine, or nakedness, or peril, or sword? But in all these things we overwhelmingly conquer through Him who loved us." Go ahead and add cancer to Paul's list. Through Christ's love, we can overwhelmingly conquer cancer as well.

Now, admittedly, there were several times during my battle with Stage IV metastatic melanoma when I sunk well below the surface of the water. Thank God I discovered Peter's backup plan as I was learning to walk above my circumstances. Whenever I began slipping down into despair, I called out to Him, and His outstretched hand took hold of mine and lifted me back up. Walk on!

♡

*Lord, teach us to keep our eyes fixed on You and not our problems.
We thank You that You catch us when we slip.*

Star Maker

joe fornear

To whom then will you liken Me that I would be his equal?" says the Holy One.
Lift up your eyes on high and see who has created these stars, The One who leads forth their host
by number, He calls them all by name; Because of the greatness of His might
and the strength of His power, not one of them is missing.

Isaiah 40:25-26

When Isaiah recorded these words of God, he knew the stars were numerous and beautiful. Little did he know the true scale of the vastness of the heavens. Astronomers tell us there are 200 billion stars residing in just one of the smaller galaxies, the Milky Way. The universe holds a mere 3,000,000,000,000,000,000 stars! That's three thousand million billion stars, each of which God has assigned a name. I suppose remembering so many names is easy compared to creating them in the first place.

The sheer volume of stars boggles the brain, but their beauty is equally astounding. We are just beginning to capture images of what God has fashioned in the far corners of the universe. There are amazing formations of gas, dust and stars which we call nebulae. Do yourself a favor and take a moment to find images of nebulae. Allow "the greatness of His might and the strength of His power" to sink in.

Is it any wonder that in hard times, God asks us to look away from our earthly dilemmas and look up to Him and His stellar handiwork? Still, how does this help if we're sick and lying flat on our backs?

In May 2003, when I was battling Stage IV metastatic melanoma, I remember lying in a hospital bed, shaken by doubts and fears which had broad-sided me in the wee hours of the night. As the Lord began redirecting my focus, He reminded me of the complexity and vastness of His creation, and how awesome He is to create such wonders. Out of nothing, He designed and launched this entire universe! Still Psalm 139:17–18 tells us He thinks of you and me constantly *and* with great fondness. Romans 8:28 says He works *all* things to the good for those who love Him.

So what is there to fear? The Star Maker loves us!

Lord, give us just a glimpse of Your true nature and we will be lifted out of our troubles.

Panic Is a Choice
joe fornear

*No temptation has overtaken you but such as is common to man; and God is faithful,
who will not allow you to be tempted beyond what you are able, but with the temptation
will provide the way of escape also, so that you will be able to endure it.*
1 Corinthians 10:13

Temptation always abounds, even when you're sick. When we're weak and vulnerable, a common temptation is to be overwhelmed by fear and doubts. In the midst of pain, bad news or a poor prognosis, panic is never far off, but neither is the way of escape. Fortunately for us, being overwhelmed is a choice and not inevitable. So how do we overcome the temptation to be gripped by fear and not the Lord's peace?

Realize you're not alone. "No temptation has overtaken you but such as is common to man." Any situation you will ever be in, another human has already been there, and managed to stand firm. You too can get through anything the Lord allows in your life.

Remember God's commitment to help you overcome. "God is faithful." You can count on Him to give you all of the coping power you need. He will never let you down.

Rest in His control. "The Lord will not allow you to be tempted beyond what you are able." When You're the absolute Master of the Universe, You can monitor and ease the difficulties of your beloved children. Praise to the Lord for that!

Remain steadfast in the face of the temptation. "With the temptation He will provide the way of escape also, so that you will be able to endure it. ..." Don't stumble over the false expectation that victory only comes through the Lord removing the temptation. He may not remove it; He might ask you to endure its presence. Either way, He will provide a way of escape through His Presence. Look for His escape route. It could come in the form of a Scripture verse, a surprise appearance from a long-lost friend, a timely financial gift or a word of comfort He speaks directly to your spirit.

We have a loving God and Creator. He does not abandon us when we need Him most! Turn your gaze to Him and not your storm.

Lord, we thank You in advance for providing everything we need to be at rest in any situation.

MIRACLES
for
TODAY

♡

Getting People's Hopes Up
joe fornear

*These signs will accompany those who have believed: in My name they will cast out demons,
they will speak with new tongues; they will pick up serpents, and if they drink any deadly poison,
it will not hurt them; they will lay hands on the sick, and they will recover.*

Mark 16:16-17

God does miracles every day, and He is absolutely delighted when we diligently seek Him for a miracle. This may surprise you, but some Bible believers would disagree with this statement. Once after I spoke about Stronghold Ministry's desire to see more healing miracles today, a Christian doctor who is experienced in both the Bible and oncology took me aside and said, "You're getting people's hopes up; you should just be getting them ready to die." I replied, "Why can't I do both?" As one who was given days to live in 2003, I assure you, I would rather have died with the hope than live without the hope of a miracle.

As cancer spread from under my arm to many sensitive sites, like my lung, kidney, stomach and pancreas, the thought hit me, Stage IV cancer is as easy for God to heal as Stage I. Jesus put it plainly, "Nothing is impossible with God." If He didn't intend to get our hopes up with that statement, may I say humbly, He sure needs a lesson on managing other's expectations.

Some fail to pursue a miraculous healing because they predetermine that God probably won't answer. Now I don't believe He guarantees healing, but I'm confident He delights when our hopes are high. I assume He continually commands us to persevere in prayer because our prayers make a tangible difference. But don't take my word for it, God says through James, "The effective prayer of a righteous man can accomplish much" (James 5:16).

My Jewish oncologist told me his patients who "beat the odds" were overwhelmingly hope-filled, Christian people who boldly sought Jesus for a miracle. Granted, this is not statistical "proof," but one should not discount such an observation from a doctor who works daily on the front lines of oncology. So go ahead and get your hopes up!

Oh, on being ready to die, do yourself a big favor, and make sure you consider the options. Eventually, whether we are healed now or not, we will die and stand before God to give an account for our lives. So to help you prepare for that moment, I encourage you to take a moment to read, "The Two Ways to Get to Heaven" in Appendix I of this book. There is much hope for now and eternity!

Lord, strengthen our faith in Your ability and willingness to do miracles in our lives.

Power Shortage Resolved

joe fornear

We have this treasure in earthen vessels, so that the surpassing greatness of the power will be of God and not from ourselves; we are afflicted in every way, but not crushed; perplexed, but not despairing; persecuted, but not forsaken; struck down, but not destroyed.

2 Corinthians 4:7–9

Coping with cancer is not hard—it is impossible. At some point during a major battle with cancer, most patients and caretakers find themselves at the end of their natural strength. Have you experienced that yet—being physically and mentally drained and exhausted? Well, don't give up; helplessness is a necessary step to being filled with "the surpassing greatness" of His power.

Notice the previous verse to our passage above. 2 Corinthians 4:6 says, "For God, who said, 'Light shall shine out of darkness,' is the One who has shone in our hearts to give the Light of the knowledge of the glory of God in the face of Christ." God's light will shine through us to this dark world if we tap into the source of true light—God Himself. Our physical body might be afflicted and crushed, but we need not despair, because this is God's way to unveil His amazing treasure within us. As we draw strength and courage from Him, He will glow through us. He is the treasure!

Our power has been spent for a reason. Let's make the shift to conscious dependence on Him, living off and depending on His power. This concept helps me make much more sense of my suffering. How about you?

Lord, encourage us that our outward breaking is for Your inward power.

♡

Help Our Unbelief!

joe fornear

And He asked his father, "How long has this been happening to him?" And he said,
"From childhood. It has often thrown him both into the fire and into the water to destroy him.
But if You can do anything, take pity on us and help us!"
And Jesus said to him, "'If You can?' All things are possible to him who believes."
Immediately the boy's father cried out and said, "I do believe; help my unbelief."
Therefore I say to you, all things for which you pray and ask,
believe that you have received them, and they will be granted you.

Mark 9:21-24

Why should we make such a big deal of faith? Simply because Jesus Christ made a big deal of faith. One moment He was rebuking someone for their lack of faith, the next moment He was extolling someone's outrageous request. It's hard to believe these faith lessons have no bearing on our prayers today! If we can't bring our impossible situations to the all-powerful, living Christ, then where can we go?

And there is good news for us who "have our doubts." Our faith does not have to be airtight to receive affirmative answers. In the gospel of Mark, a man received a miracle while utilizing less than perfect faith. He approached Jesus for his son, who had been possessed by a destructive evil spirit. He pleaded, "If You can do anything, take pity on us and help us!" (Mark 9:22).

In Jesus' response, He is not only stating that He (Jesus) can do anything, He asserts that the man can also get amazing results through faith. Jesus is teaching the man to believe his prayer will come to pass. The man realized Jesus was making his own faith the issue. So Mark tells us, "Immediately the boy's father cried out and said, 'I do believe; help my unbelief.'" Jesus had just rebuked His disciples for their inability to cast out the demon. He declared their unbelief as the reason they were not heard. "O unbelieving generation, how long shall I be with you? How long shall I put up with you? Bring him to Me!" (Mark 9:18–19).

Jesus is intending to teach us how to pray. Let's learn His secrets of praying effectively. Let's ask Him and trust Him to help chase away our unbelief. Then leave the results to our Sovereign God. Be bold. Amen?

Lord, we believe. Dispel our unbelief. Take us to new levels of trust and prayer with You.

The Only Way to Pray

joe fornear

And Jesus answered saying to them, "Have faith in God. Truly I say to you, whoever says to this mountain, 'Be taken up and cast into the sea,' and does not doubt in his heart, but believes that what he says is going to happen, it will be granted him. Therefore I say to you, all things for which you pray and ask, believe that you have received them, and they will be granted you."

Mark 11:22-24

If understanding prayer is like a doctoral degree, then frankly, I'm still in kindergarten. Yet maybe child-like faith is in order when it comes to prayer. I'm convinced we overanalyze Jesus' lessons on prayer. They are to be applied zealously today, but instead we qualify His instructions until we strip away His plain meaning. We mean well; we are trying to prepare ourselves and others for unanswered prayers. So we talk ourselves out of wanting anything. *"God will probably not answer this request, so I need to pray in a way that accounts for the difficulty of this situation."* Then we proceed to pray in a manner that strips an essential ingredient from our prayers—faith.

According to Jesus, there is only one way to pray—with faith. He said, "Therefore I say to you, all things for which you pray and ask, believe that you have received them, and they will be granted you" (Mark 11:21–24). Note that Jesus does not hedge on or account for the relative difficulty of our requests. He commands us to pray with faith for "all things" we ask, whether our requests are large or small. In the previous verses, He concluded we could move mountains with faith. After making our requests, we should simply follow His command and believe we have *already* received our request. Don't disobey the Lord by entertaining all of the "buts" that undermine this clear instruction. Just do what He says!

Praying with faith is "the only way to pray." In James 1:5–8, James is very dogmatic about the importance of praying with faith. Wisdom from God is the prayer request:

But if any of you lacks wisdom, let him ask of God, who gives to all generously and without reproach, and it will be given to him. But he must ask in faith without any doubting, for the one who doubts is like the surf of the sea, driven and tossed by the wind. For that man ought not to expect that he will receive anything from the Lord, being a double-minded man, unstable in all his ways (James 1:5–8).

Do you pray with faith as James and Jesus commanded? We are not tasked with figuring out the overall agenda of God. Let's just perform our role as He has directed! Successful sports teams are made up of personnel who fill various roles. As each player carries out their role at the direction of the coach, the team succeeds. The same is true in following our Coach in our role in prayer. We should simply do our part and pray with faith, believing we already have our request. We don't need to understand everything about prayer; we should be childlike and just believe. God will figure out the rest. Amen?

Lord, help us to simply follow your ways and not seek to figure everything out.

changing God's Mind

joe fornear

So the LORD changed His mind about the harm which He said He would do to His people.
Exodus 32:14

Some may wonder about prayer, "If God already knows whether He will answer or not, why even bother to pray? It won't make any difference. He already knows what He will do." No, no, a thousand times, no! In the Scriptures, there are amazing exchanges between God and men when prayer not only makes a difference, it appears to even "change" God's mind!

In the book of Exodus, after Israel's repeated rebellion, the Lord vehemently declared His decision to destroy the people of Israel. He even announced a new plan to make a nation from Moses as the new head. But Moses interceded for them and his prayers evidently made a big difference. "So the LORD changed His mind about the harm which He said He would do to His people" (Exodus 32:14). I think we are way too passive in our prayers, don't you?

There is another notable occasion when God declared that King Hezekiah would die from a serious illness.

In those days Hezekiah became mortally ill. And Isaiah the prophet the son of Amoz came to him and said to him, "Thus says the LORD, 'Set your house in order, for you shall die and not live'" (2 Kings 20:1).

After delivering God's will, His verdict, Isaiah then left to go home. But after hearing of his fate, Hezekiah prayed earnestly and his fervent prayers "changed" God's mind. "I have heard your prayer, I have seen your tears; behold, I will heal you. On the third day you shall go up to the house of the LORD. I will add fifteen years to your life" (2 Kings 20:5–6). God changed His mind here as well.

Certainly God knew when He made these pronouncements that He would eventually change His mind. Perhaps He was just testing His follower's passion for prayer? I don't believe our prayers are guaranteed to be answered, but I'm determined to discover the limits of the mysterious power of prayer. Won't you join me?

♡

Lord, please give us mighty endurance and power in prayer.

Increase Our Faith

joe fornear

Then the disciples came to Jesus privately and said, "Why could we not drive it out?"
And He said to them, "Because of the littleness of your faith; for truly I say to you,
if you have faith the size of a mustard seed, you will say to this mountain,
'Move from here to there,' and it will move; and nothing will be impossible to you.

Matthew 17:19-20

Can the size of our faith make a difference in God answering our prayers? Absolutely yes! Jesus says so in Matthew 17:19. The disciples' prayers to cast out a demon went unanswered because of the "littleness of their faith." So let's take the time to spark each other's faith. God delights in showing off His power in response to our prayers of faith.

I have, however, observed prayer warriors with greater faith than mine who did not receive a miracle healing. So I'm not suggesting if one has enough faith they are guaranteed healing. We don't control God with our prayers. One champion of the faith, the Apostle Paul, prayed diligently for God to remove a series of severe hardships, which he called a "thorn in the flesh." It was later revealed to him that the thorn would remain in order to keep him humble. This situation and other similar Bible lessons teach that God has a Higher Purpose when He doesn't answer our faith-filled prayers. Still, why would Jesus stress praying with faith and with boldness if they did not matter?

In the context of Matthew 17, mountains are symbolic of the humanly impossible situations in our lives. When we're in a bind, Jesus must be pleased that we are drawn to passages on moving mountains. The good news is our faith does not need to be that big for Him to answer the prayer. He said faith the size of a mere mustard seed can move mountains. Mustard seeds are small, about the size of the ball in a ballpoint pen. This is just enough faith to move Him to activate His powers and abilities. Mountains *can* be moved.

Lord, You are the author and perfecter of our faith, please increase our faith!

Hometown Jesus

joe fornear

He came to His hometown and began teaching them in their synagogue, so that they
were astonished, and said, "Where did this man get this wisdom and these miraculous powers?
Is not this the carpenter's son? Is not His mother called Mary, and His brothers, James
and Joseph and Simon and Judas? And His sisters, are they not all with us?
Where then did this man get all these things?" And they took offense at Him. But Jesus said to them,
"A prophet is not without honor except in his hometown and in his own household."
And He did not do many miracles there because of their unbelief.

Matthew 13:54-58

They say familiarity breeds contempt. In this passage from Matthew, Jesus basically confirms that dynamic. The people of His hometown knew much about Him, perhaps too much. They shared a long history, and because that history did not include miracles, they determined it never would. They had heard the amazing stories, yet refused to believe God might work among them in new ways. Sadly, their expectations were fully met. Little expected of God; little received from God.

This leads to a penetrating question for us. Have we limited the work of God in our own lives? Perhaps there's a reason miracles are few—or missing altogether! Someone might respond, "How could we even know on this side of heaven?" It is true the Lord's ways are mysterious and beyond our manipulation or control. Yet hopefully Jesus' famous phrase will never be used of us, "Oh you of little faith." Will He say to us in the end, "I was willing to do so much more for you"?

God wants to show off His power over some of man's most difficult obstacles —like cancer. I don't believe we are guaranteed miracles, but certainly we should ask for one! "You do not have because you do not ask" (James 4:2). So I encourage you to gather your loved ones together. Read several passages on His challenges to us to pray. Ask and *believe* Him for miracles. Then watch what He will do!

♡

Lord, if You choose not to heal, help us submit to that,
but we want to trust You for a miracle in our life!

Cry Out to the One Who Heals

joe fornear

In those days Hezekiah became ill and was at the point of death.
The prophet Isaiah son of Amoz went to him and said, "This is what the LORD says:
Put your house in order, because you are going to die; you will not recover."
Hezekiah turned his face to the wall and prayed to the LORD, "Remember, O LORD, how I have
walked before you faithfully and with wholehearted devotion and have done
what is good in your eyes." And Hezekiah wept bitterly.
Before Isaiah had left the middle court, the word of the LORD came to him:
"Go back and tell Hezekiah, the leader of my people, 'This is what the LORD, the God of your father
David, says: I have heard your prayer and seen your tears; I will heal you.'"

2 Kings 20:1-5

At the point of death, God mercifully extended Hezekiah's life for 15 years. Certainly his heartfelt prayers made a deep impression on God. Granted, God doesn't answer all such prayers, but He often intervenes in dramatic fashion.

As long as there are serious illnesses, there will be cries for healing. As long as there are cries for healing, there will be miraculous interventions by the Lord. As long as I have breath, I will encourage the hurting to seek God's miraculous intervention in their lives. People often report to Stronghold Ministry how the Lord healed them when they were at the point of death, extending their lives for years, just as He did for Hezekiah—and just as He did for me. We have shared many of their stories in our newsletters.

I am convinced that God wants to intervene more than we think. May He grant us that small, mustard-seed-sized faith to pursue Him for the impossible. God loves to defy human odds!

♡

Lord, we know and believe You can and want to perform miracles. Please work a miracle in my life.

VICTORY MARCH
in the
WILDERNESS

♡

Victory March in the Wilderness Part 1

joe fornear

O God, when You went forth before Your people, when You marched through the wilderness, Selah.
The earth quaked; the heavens also dropped rain at the presence of God;
Sinai itself quaked at the presence of God, the God of Israel. You shed abroad a plentiful rain,
O God; You confirmed Your inheritance when it was parched.

Psalm 68:7-9

Journeying through life's deserts can be very frightening. Thankfully, the Lord reigns everywhere, including in the desert! Psalm 68 is a proclamation that the Lord provides riches in the wilderness, where David found himself in literal and figurative dilemmas. He wrote to comfort himself and his readers. If God was faithful to Israel in the wilderness, He will be faithful to David, too. And He will be faithful to us as well!

There are several fears common to travelers in the desert. Certainly one is this: Will I become lost and disoriented in the desert?

If we are fighting cancer or in some other major crisis, we travel on perilous roads. Our decisions seem to make the difference between life and death. We hope we're making the right decisions. We cry out to God to lead us. We trust He is guiding. Well, glory to God that even in the wilderness, He promises to lead. Psalm 68:7 says, He "goes forth before His people" through the wilderness. In other words, He already is out in front and leading us though the harsh conditions! The Hebrew word at the end of verse 7 is "Selah," which is an inspirational literary device. It means to pause, reflect, wonder and worship. So, Selah! We can rest—He is guiding us!

In the midst of trials, He promises to lead every step and grant us wisdom along the way. "If any of you lacks wisdom, let him ask of God, who gives to all generously and without reproach, and it will be given to him" (James 1). This verse promises that the Lord will lead when we ask and believe He will guide us. Since He is leading, there is no reason to fear any destination! Never doubt that He is leading you. Don't let your emotions overrule His word. He is faithful, just trust that He is leading you and don't fear navigating through the desert.

Lord, we know you care deeply, so we trust You to guide us through this wilderness time in our lives.

Victory March in the Wilderness Part 2

joe fornear

O God, when You went forth before Your people, when You marched through the wilderness, Selah.
The earth quaked; the heavens also dropped rain at the presence of God;
Sinai itself quaked at the presence of God, the God of Israel. You shed abroad a plentiful rain,
O God; You confirmed Your inheritance when it was parched.

Psalm 68:7-9

There is another common fear in the deserts of our lives: Is it possible to overcome when conditions are so harsh?

In Psalm 68, David proclaims that God "marched through the wilderness." This picture is that of a victorious king leading a parade of jubilant subjects. He is King of the glorious city filled with celebration, but He is also King of the desert places. Paul "saw" this victory march of our King as well: "He always leads us in triumphal procession in Christ" (2 Corinthians 2:14). Do you see His victory for you in your wilderness journey?

Keep in mind, Paul endured vast stretches of desert places in the form of cruel persecutions and constant sufferings. He was whipped, beaten, betrayed, stoned and imprisoned. Like Paul, our bodies and emotions may be banged up and bruised because of illness or trials. Yet he rose above all of his circumstances. His secret: "I can do all things through Christ, who strengthens me" (Philippians 4:13).

Though we *have* physical bodies, we *are* spiritual beings who overcome through the supernatural strengthening of our spirits. "Therefore we do not lose heart, but though our outer man is decaying, yet our inner man is being renewed day by day" (2 Corinthians 4:16). Even if your body is weakening, let Him strengthen your inner person. Ask Him to open your eyes to the reality of His victory in the wilderness. God is our Stronghold!

♡

Lord, even when our bodies are weak, You lead us in victorious procession in spiritual realms.

Victory March in the Wilderness
Part 3

joe fornear

O God, when You went forth before Your people, when You marched through the wilderness, Selah.
The earth quaked; the heavens also dropped rain at the presence of God;
Sinai itself quaked at the presence of God, the God of Israel. You shed abroad a plentiful rain,
O God; You confirmed Your inheritance when it was parched.

Psalm 68:7-9

Deserts are no match for our victorious King! Yet we don't always stand firm in that knowledge. Another common fear in the desert is this: "Will there be sufficient provisions, like water and food?" In other words, "Do I have enough resources to handle my wilderness journey?" Desert travelers are often loaded down with worries, and many of our "what-if" questions revolve around resources.

Spiritual Resources. "What if I come to the end of my strength will I be able to cope?"

Material Resources. "Will I—will we—will they have enough money?"

Relational Resources. "What will my kids miss out on while I'm sick?"

Psalm 68:9 reminds us that God "confirmed His inheritance when it was parched." We may run out of resources, but He never does. No matter how horrible our conditions, His inheritance and resources will be sufficient. Don't let pain, stress or bad news cause you to panic. Simply rest in Him and trust Him for everything you or your loved ones need. He is committed to take care of every concern you have. Twice this passage stresses that His "presence" provides a "rain," even "plentiful rain." He will provide!

During my brutal cancer fight with Stage IV metastatic melanoma, there were several times I feared running out of strength, money and energy to raise my kids, but my anxiety was unnecessary. When I really needed something,

He was there. I'm not saying it was easy to cope; it was very difficult, but His presence and inheritance made the journey so much more manageable. Many times, He even made the journey pleasant. Drink the rain!

Lord, we thank You that we can trust that Your inheritance is vast and plentiful!

Carried Out of the Desert
terri fornear

Let his left hand be under my head and his right hand embrace me … who is this
coming up from the wilderness leaning on her beloved?
Song of Songs 8:3 & 5

I love the late summer weather in Texas. Some plants actually start blooming instead of wilting even after months of extreme heat. The buds peek out, hoping rain and cooler air will allow them to blossom.

Recently, while coming out of my own dry season, I felt afraid I would lean on those blessings too hard and they would disappear. Joe is playing basketball again after more than two years of missing out because of neck and back issues. My son Jesse has found a job he loves after months of searching. My daughter Amy has graduated from college. God has been good through this heat wave, but I haven't always believed in His goodness, I was often just hoping.

Then I read in The Song of Songs in 8:3 and 5, "Let his left hand be under my head and his right hand embrace me." And, "Who is this coming up from the wilderness, leaning on her beloved?" I see myself learning to walk out of the wilderness, feeling His right hand embracing me (Jesus is at the right hand of the Father, as we know from Ephesians 1:20). Letting His left hand hold my head up, I look Him in the eyes. (Fixing my eyes on Jesus, the author and finisher of my faith—Hebrews 12:2). I learn to lean on my Beloved for the next steps in my life.

Some days it is easy to see and feel His hold on me. On other hot, dry days, I have to just believe He has His hold on me. May this be a day that you believe and feel that He is embracing you and leading you out of the desert.

Lord, we want to trust You when times are tough and also when they are good.

HEAVEN, DEATH
and the
RESURRECTION

♡

Victory Guaranteed

joe fornear

Our citizenship is in heaven. He will transform the body of our humble state into conformity with the body of His glory, by the exertion of the power that He has even to subject all things to Himself.

Philippians 3:20-21

Do you ever just "hope" the Lord knows what He is doing? We are told that His ways are not our ways (Isaiah 55:9), but sometimes our journey can seem so long and difficult, even pointless.

Consider the children of Israel at Jericho. How many times did they circle the city before the walls fell down? Did you answer, "Seven"? I read recently that the answer is actually 13, because on the seventh day, they circled seven times, for a total of 13 laps (Joshua 6:15). I mention this only because the additional laps add to the oddity of the situation.

At points during this journey, the Israelites probably thought, or said, "This is dumb. Why do we have to keep circling this city? God could knock these walls down with a snap of His finger. Haven't we walked long enough?"

I think there is a takeaway lesson here for followers of Christ who are fighting cancer. As your lap count increases, you may grow weary, but you can trust the walls will eventually fall. Absolute victory is guaranteed in Christ. His Resurrection demonstrates for all time the incredible scope of His deliverance. Even if He heals me a hundred times in this life, someday I will take my final lap. But praise to the Lord God Almighty, it will be a victory lap!

Paul said it like this, "Our citizenship is in heaven. He will transform the body of our humble state into conformity with the body of His glory, by the exertion of the power that He has even to subject all things to Himself" (Philippians 3:20–21). Can anyone use a transformed body? In His Word, the Bible, He has written this promise of victory. He grants it to those who simply cling to forgiveness of their sins through Jesus Christ's substitutionary death on the cross.

If you're exhausted from circling what seems like an endless city, remember to lean on Him. He will carry you to victory! You will eventually step over crumpled walls! Your journey is never in vain. Victory is guaranteed!

Lord, help us stand on Your many promises of absolute and total victory in the end.

Fear NO Evil

joe fornear

Therefore, since the children share in flesh and blood, He Himself likewise also partook of the same,
that through death He might render powerless him who had the power of death, that is,
the devil, and might free those who through fear of death were subject to slavery all their lives.

Hebrews 2:14-15

It may not be pleasant, but it is always wise to face fears. With God on our side, even the fear of death is conquered through Jesus Christ! Jesus took on a human body, tasted death Himself and returned to prove His dominance over man's ultimate enemy. So if and whenever we walk through that valley of death's shadow, we need fear no evil.

When diagnosed with cancer, many are unnerved by how their battle might end. With some cancers, doctors often make predictions about our longevity —eight months; two months. In May 2003, I was told I had just days to live. Masses growing on the head and tail of my pancreas had locked up the pancreatic ducts, and Stage IV melanoma had spread to multiple sites, including other vital organs, my lung and kidney.

So I looked death square in the eye, and marched forward without a single doubt. Well, not quite. I had always fancied myself so full of faith, but for two very long days, the foundations of my faith were rattled by fear of the unknown. How bad could my condition get? I was humbled to realize my trust had been in my own courage and resources, and those resources had run dry. I had thought I could handle anything, as I was very tough, you see.

Yet true to His nature, God, our Stronghold, held me up during my wavering. I looked to Him in my weakness and I became strong as He provided supernatural resources to cope with dying. He infused me with confidence that His grace would match any trauma of my final days. He promised me grace to die; you might call it "dying grace." Then I found myself not only prepared to die, but eager to die. I could echo what Paul wrote in Philippians 1: 21, "For to me, to live is Christ and to die is gain."

For now, He obviously still has work for me to do. Yet I learned an invaluable lesson for my future. Hebrews 2:15 reveals the source of fears of death—the devil—an evil, spiritual being. Like it or not, we are engaged in an invisible spiritual battle, which is heightened, of course, by life-threatening diseases such as cancer. Yet the devil's power is dwarfed by the Lord's awesome power! The Lord carries us through any struggle, including everyday problems, relational conflicts, even a rough cancer fight. Certainly He will usher us gently through that final gate to everlasting life.

If you have a life-threatening cancer, we fervently pray He will heal you to live a long, abundant life! Yet eventually we'll all leave this earthly realm. That, too, is a grace in itself, as who wants to live here forever? If you feel your time is drawing near, be unflinchingly courageous in Him, knowing He will carry you each step of the way. God is good, thus, He has a plan for everything.

You may wonder how I can be so sure that God will welcome me into heaven. For more, read Appendix I, "The Two Ways to Get to Heaven."

Lord, we thank You that You give us abundant grace for every step of our journeys,
even the final ones.

Your Resurrection Day

joe fornear

Therefore, being always of good courage, and knowing that while we are at home in the body
we are absent from the Lord—for we walk by faith, not by sight—we are of good courage,
I say, and prefer rather to be absent from the body and to be at home with the Lord.

2 Corinthians 5:6-8

When I was battling cancer, there was a topic that frequently crossed my mind, but I did not want to discuss it. Frankly, I did not appreciate it when others raised the issue with my wife or me. We were so deep into survival mode; the last thing I wanted to talk about was the d-word—death. Yet I knew I was fighting for my life.

Pausing to consider that I might not make it seemed counterproductive. Entertaining the possibility of dying might weaken my resolve to live. Yet Solomon, the wisest man who ever walked the earth, except Jesus, taught us a contrary approach regarding death. "It is better to go to a house of mourning than a house of feasting, for that is the end of all men; and the living will take it to heart" (Ecclesiastes 7:2). Solomon suggested that whether we live 70 more years, or 70 more hours, we should be preparing for the next life, and living each day as though it was our last. Death doesn't go away because we refuse to think about it.

Jesus often attempted to prepare His followers for His departure. He told them He would be beaten and crucified. He also taught them that He would rise; that ultimately death would not have the last word. Later, Paul extended Christ's victory to us! "Christ is the first fruits, after that, at His second coming, those who are Christ's will also rise" (1 Corinthians 15:23). So Jesus' resurrection is actually a foretaste of our own resurrection from the dead—that is, if we truly belong to Christ.

Now I am definitely not suggesting anyone give up on their fight. No way! But I am saying that the Resurrection helps us lose our fear of dying, so that we can face it square in the eye, and proclaim with Paul, "Oh death, where is your victory? Oh death, where is your sting" (1 Corinthians 15:55).

♡

Thank You, Lord, for Christ's rising, as it means we too will rise!

Moving the Largest Stone
joe fornear

As it began to dawn toward the first day of the week, Mary Magdalene and the other Mary
came to look at the grave. And behold, a severe earthquake had occurred,
for an angel of the Lord descended from heaven and came and rolled away the stone and sat upon it.
Matthew 28:1-2

At five feet in diameter, this stone was huge, but it was still just a rock. Several men could move it. These days man and his machines can literally move a mountain. We have created space ships to zoom to the moon to retrieve its rocks. Yet man cannot prevent becoming part of the rocks himself. Eventually death picks us off, one by one. Why is talking about death so uncomfortable to many? Probably because it makes us feel so helpless.

I once witnessed a fatal motorcycle accident. I don't think I ever felt so helpless. A car turned in front of a fast moving motorcycle and the cycle slid and hit the car very, very hard. I ran to the driver who was separated from his bike. He was quite young. I heard later he was only 23 years old. By the time I came to his side, his blood was flowing like a tiny river down the street. I tried in vain to communicate with him. I prayed. A doctor passed by and jumped out of her car. She frantically pumped the man's chest. She stopped, felt his pulse, looked at me and shook her head. A policeman rushed over, and for a few moments administered mouth to mouth resuscitation, to no avail. Soon paramedics were swarming, and I moved aside. Futile attempts were made to revive the man with oxygen tanks and shock paddles. Soon all stopped trying. In this case, all of man's best efforts fell short. Doctors, policemen, paramedics—none made any difference.

The young man's girlfriend approached the scene. She had been waiting for his arrival just one block from the accident. After the impact, his motorcycle had skidded and propelled itself an entire block and stopped right in front of her apartment. She was rattled, but still hopeful. She kept insisting there must be a chance. Denial and disbelief reigned; she would not give in to the finality of it all without a fight. I understood. Death is brutal to loved ones, and sometimes there is no warning. I still find myself grieving for the man, but also grieving my own helplessness. I knew intellectually I couldn't prevent what happened, but the experience drove the point uncomfortably deep.

Fortunately, there is a mighty One who can indeed overcome death! Through the Resurrection of Jesus Christ, God provided the way to conquer man's ultimate foe. Though death will visit each of us, it will be trumped by our own resurrection, if we are in relationship with Christ through faith. "Christ the first fruits, after that those who are Christ's at His coming will also rise" (1 Corinthians 15:23).

Through sheer might He has cast aside the greatest boulder that had once blocked man's passage into eternal life. In Jesus Christ, on that first Easter morning, God demonstrated His power to deliver us from death. I praise Him that He is more formidable than our worst problem. Now imagine what He can do with all those little problems we have? "Oh death, where is thy sting?" (Romans 15:55).

Lord, strengthen our confidence in You, as You have overcome every foe by displaying even Your power over death in the Resurrection of Jesus from the grave.

The Win-Win of the Resurrection

joe fornear

Fixing our eyes on Jesus, the author and perfecter of faith, who for the joy set before Him endured the cross, despising the shame, and has sat down at the right hand of the throne of God.

Hebrews 12:2

I recently read of a patient fighting advanced cancer who said he was in a "win-win" position. "If God heals me, I'll be so happy. If He doesn't, I'll go to heaven, which is even better." Even at 14 years old, this young man had a firm grasp on the amazing power of Almighty God. The Lord can certainly heal any disease, and He can certainly raise us up from the dead. So we can trust Him either way. This is the abiding message of the Resurrection of Jesus Christ.

Jesus set the example for this win-win approach to life—and death. Hebrews 12:2 tells us He endured the cross because He knew the joy which awaited Him in heaven. This is why Hebrews tells us "to fix our eyes on Jesus." He not only models the attitude we hope to have in the face of death, He gives us the ability to develop and display that attitude.

Yet how can anyone be certain they will go to heaven? The Bible says we enter this win-win state the moment we receive Jesus Christ as our personal Savior. He promises to give the free gift of heaven to those who do just one thing—believe. For more, see Appendix I, "The Two Ways to Get to Heaven."

A win-win resurrection perspective frees us from destructive feelings and thoughts. Fear and anxiety loosen their hold when we entrust our lives into God's hands. One thing is for certain, we will all eventually be healed!

Lord, we know because of the Resurrection, our battle will ultimately end in eternal victory.

PRAYER
and
FAITH

♡

Wake up Call—To Grace

joe fornear

So then, does He who provides you with the Spirit and works miracles among you,
do it by the works of the Law, or by hearing with faith?

Galatians 3:5

A "wake up call" is any circumstance that triggers reexamination and re-alignment of our priorities. Being diagnosed with cancer surely woke me up, and definitely got my attention. The scary news and the ferocity of the battle rattled the foundations of my faith.

There is an old, wise saying, "We don't usually change when we see the light; we change when we feel the heat." As I passed through the blaze of aggressive cancer and treatments, I cried out to God for relief. What must I do to be healed? I was ready to make changes and sacrifice for Him. Ironically, His response was not for me to be more holy; to spend more time with Him; to search myself for some deep, dark sin. I should simply seek Him for undeserved blessings. There was nothing I could do to make myself worthy of His healing touch. I woke up—to grace.

The author of Hebrews encourages us to boldly and confidently approach God for this undeserved help. "Therefore let us draw near with confidence to the throne of grace, so that we may receive mercy and find grace to help in time of need" (Hebrews 4:16).

Galatians 3:5 stresses the Lord works on the basis of grace through faith. We should not try to somehow *earn* His blessings. We can boldly approach God through Jesus' perfectly righteous life, not our own righteousness. Jesus' death on the cross washed away my sins through faith, enabling the Father to pour out *free* blessings on me, including physical healing from cancer.

While trying to grasp the depths of this grace, several points became clear to me. I should:

- Resist the notion that God owes me anything.

- Refrain from making deals or promises to entice God to answer me.
- Readily admit and confess my past and present failings.
- Refuse to dwell on my past sins, since they're forgiven in Christ.
- Realize I don't have to pay Him back for His blessings. How could I ever repay Him?

If we pray right and have enough faith, is God guaranteed to heal? No. Yet our best appeal to Him is through His grace. So let your crisis wake you up—to grace.

Lord, we don't ask for healing and comfort because of our goodness,
but we approach You through Your grace alone.

In the Prayer Closet

terri fornear

No longer do I call you slaves, for the slave does not know what his master is doing; but I have called you friends, for all things that I have heard from My Father I have made known to you.

John 15:15

(Terri wrote these thoughts to her church in February 2003. At this time, Joe had already undergone three surgeries to remove Stage IV metastatic melanoma. He was out of town for lengthy interleuken-2 treatments in Pittsburgh, while Terri stayed in Dallas to care for their teenagers, Jesse and Amy.)

Prayer has been one of those Christian activities that I've been wrestling with this year. I first had to confess to God that I didn't think it mattered what I asked. He ultimately does things His way. I realized this was an attitude of angry surrender. Then I asked Him to teach me to pray with an attitude of servant surrender. His disciples asked this, so it was the "spiritual" thing to do.

This was the beginning of God breaking my heart to see His heart. My heart had been angry, hurt and very resentful in the last few years. A hardened heart.

I began to pray for jobs for others; for health for others. I prayed for *others*. That was safer; I did not have to face the answers so personally. If the prayers were not answered, I had nothing to risk. It was easier to accept a "no" for someone else's request. God was "safe" this way, too. He was off the hook, and I could still do a spiritual thing and feel good about myself.

There was only one "problem." He was hearing and answering my prayers! He cared that I was talking to Him about my heart's desires for others. He was knocking down my self-protective wall against Him. He was asking me to be His friend, not His slave. He reminded me of a verse in John 15:15, "No longer do I call you slaves, for the slave does not know what his master is doing; but I have called you friends, for all things that I have heard from My Father I have made known to you." He wanted to share His heart with me. He wanted to tell me what He was doing!

I had been depending on my friends. I have great friends. I could list their names, and tell you how they have been a great gift to me. My friends were doing a good job; I did not need God to be my friend. They were His children, so His friendship came through them. I can see them and that was good enough. Still, God wants my friendship. He wants me to know His heart and to see Him from a heavenly point of view. Most of all He wants me to hear from Him. Prayer has taken a new bend for me. I'm just beginning a journey that I know little about, except that He is on the other end sharing His life with me.

This storm of "cancer" in our home has been interesting. I cannot put words to it. Tears seem to be its primary language; a language He is sharing with me so intimately. I know He "hears" each one of them.

Because of your prayers, your faith and your love for me and my family, you are His face to me throughout the day. I have a fear and trembling kind of excitement about what God is doing in our church, in my family and in my heart. Yet, it's a good fear; knowing God has great love for me and purpose for this storm. He is definitely in the boat with me—with us.

Lord, open our hearts to your love, that we would know your friendship,
and know what you are doing in our lives.

Amazing Jesus

terri fornear

Now when Jesus heard this, He marveled and said to those who were following,
"Truly I say to you, I have not found such great faith with anyone in Israel.

Matthew 8:10

But she said, "Yes, Lord; but even the dogs feed on the crumbs which fall from their masters' table."
Then Jesus said to her, "O woman, your faith is great; it shall be done for you as you wish."
And her daughter was healed at once.

Matthew 15:27-28

What do you think it would take to amaze Jesus? After all, He created the entire universe! He exists in heaven and earth. He knows everything—past, present and future. Yet while on earth, there was something that truly impressed Him to the point of exclaiming, "Now that's really something! Wow!"

Never in the four gospels was He astounded by anyone's:

- Righteousness
- Great gifts
- Musical ability (after all, He heard angels sing daily)
- Service (He looked at Martha's service and basically said, "Something's missing.")
- Education
- Knowledge (He never said to Matthew, "You're so smart, your financial ability is incredible!")

Jesus was amazed by just one thing—faith.

- The Roman Centurion: "Just say the Word ..." (Matthew 8:8–10).
- The Canaanite woman: "Even the dogs get crumbs ..." (Matthew 15:27–28).

Actually, He was also amazed at the lack of faith in His hometown, Nazareth (Mark 6:6).

The work of God is believing. Consider the work of faith of the men and women in the Bible. This "cloud of witnesses" is looking down at the fruits of their labor in you and me.

They were stoned, they were sawn in two, they were tempted, they were put to death with the sword; they went about in sheepskins, in goatskins, being destitute, afflicted, ill-treated (men of whom the world was not worthy), wandering in deserts and mountains and caves and holes in the ground. And all these, having gained approval through their faith, did not receive what was promised, because God had provided something better for us. (Hebrews 11:37–40).

These believers amazed Jesus. Their hard-working faith has been passed down, so now we, too, can amaze Jesus and experience the *amazing* Jesus.

As you live today, walk in faith. It's the quality that makes Jesus smile, and causes His heart to be in awe. It's the bridge to bring Jesus' life to those around us.

Lord, reveal Your power to us that we would be amazed by You and have amazing faith in You.

More Than Enough!

joe fornear

And He has said to me, "My grace is sufficient for you, for power is perfected in weakness."
Most gladly, therefore, I will rather boast about my weaknesses, so that the power of Christ may
dwell in me. Therefore I am well content with weaknesses, with insults, with distresses,
with persecutions, with difficulties, for Christ's sake; for when I am weak, then I am strong.

2 Corinthians 12:9-10

During my battle with Stage IV metastatic melanoma, the Lord used the devotional book, *Streams in the Desert*, to encourage me and to help me to make sense of my sufferings. In one entry, there is an inspirational quote by Charles Spurgeon, a pastor from the 1800s. The gist of the quote is that God's resources are more than enough to handle any need we have. It is a powerful illustration.

The other evening I was riding home after a heavy day's work; I was wearied and depressed; and swiftly and suddenly as a lightning flash, this text laid hold of me: "My grace is sufficient for you!" (2 Corinthians 12:9). When I got home, I looked it up in the original, and finally it dawned upon me what the text was saying, MY grace is sufficient for YOU. "Why," I said to myself, "I should think it is!" and I burst out laughing.

It seemed to make unbelief so absurd. It was as though some little fish, being very thirsty, was troubled about drinking the river dry; and Father River said, "Drink away, little fish, my stream is sufficient for you!" Or as if a little mouse in the granaries of Egypt after seven years of plenty, feared lest it should die of famine, and Joseph said, "Cheer up, little mouse, my granaries are sufficient for you!" Again I imagined a man on the mountain top saying to himself, "I fear I shall exhaust all the oxygen in the atmosphere." But the earth cries, "Breathe away, O man, and fill your lungs; my atmosphere is sufficient for you!"

So drink, eat and breathe His superabundant grace to comfort, strengthen and heal you. And always remember, there is more where that came from!

♡

Lord, open our eyes to the sufficiency of Your grace, knowing Your resources could never run out.

He's In Your Corner

joe fornear

Therefore He is able also to save forever those who draw near to God through Him,
since He always lives to make intercession for them.

Hebrews 7:5

One of the many benefits of receiving Christ as our personal Savior is that we have the perfect Advocate before God the Father. We have the absolute best representation. The Bible says in the book of Hebrews that Jesus Christ is our eternal High Priest. His work as an advocate or intercessor is described in Hebrews 7:5, "He always lives to make intercession for them."

This is fantastic news when we are in a crisis, such as being diagnosed with cancer. He *lives* or exists to make intercession for us! Not only does His intercession constantly cover our sins because of His saving work on the cross, but in John 14:12–14, Jesus makes bold promises as a result of His position at the Father's right hand.

> Truly, truly, I say to you, he who believes in Me, the works that I do, he will do also; and greater works than these he will do; because I go to the Father. Whatever you ask in My name, that will I do, so that the Father may be glorified in the Son. If you ask Me anything in My name, I will do it.

Jesus "has the ear" of His Father and our Father, the Lord of the universe. He will pull some strings for us! This, my friends, is the wonderful advocacy that Jesus Christ has for us. Don't be afraid; boldly ask Him for great things. Yes, ask Him to totally heal you. We may not know exactly how He will answer, but we definitely know how He tells us to pray. We can ask Him anything! He guarantees He will give us everything we need for our journeys. He's in your corner now!

♡

Lord, inspire us to ask great things of You, that You may be glorified through answering our prayers.

PROLOGUE

♡

Can You Help Us Spread His Comfort?

joe and terri fornear

*Blessed be the God and Father of our Lord Jesus Christ, the Father of mercies
and God of all comfort, who comforts us in all our affliction so that we will be able to comfort those
who are in any affliction with the comfort with which we ourselves are comforted by God.*

2 Corinthians 1:3-4

The beauty of God's comfort is that it is transferable! Stronghold Ministry thrives on spreading the comfort we received during our cancer battle, but we could use your help. Here is how:

Pray for us. We would be honored if you would pray regularly for us. We need it!

Send us a testimony. If you are a cancer patient or a caretaker, and have been touched by Stronghold Ministry, we would love to know. With your permission we would share your story in hopes that others who don't know us will be encouraged to contact us.

Donate to the ministry. As a nonprofit organization, Stronghold relies on donations to operate. If you can help us financially we would be very grateful. To donate, go to the Donate page of our website, or send a check to Stronghold Ministry, P.O. Box 38478, Dallas, TX 75238. We are confident the Lord will bless you for helping us to help the sick. We are an IRS 501(c)3 nonprofit organization. Your donations are tax deductible in the United States.

Give us some feedback. There is always room for improvement on our part. If you have some feedback or input on how we can better serve cancer patients, please write us at jfor@mystronghold.org.

APPENDIX I

♡

The Two Ways to Get to Heaven
Are You Heaven Bound?

Ninety percent of Americans believe in heaven—and a whopping 85 percent believe they will go to heaven when they die (according to an ABC news poll on October 5, 2005). Yet how do we know for sure if we will go to heaven? This should not be a guessing matter. After all, heaven and hell last for eternity.

God Himself wants us to know *now* how to get to heaven. That is why He left us a written, objective record of His thoughts so we would not be in the dark. This record is the Bible—His Word. The apostle John stated the purpose for which he wrote, "I write to you so that you may know that you have eternal life" (1 John 5:13). So, consider now the two ways to get to heaven.

Plan A: Be perfect

If you want to be judged based on your deeds, Galatians 3:10 clearly sets out the requirements: "For as many as are of the works of the Law are under a curse; for it is written, 'Cursed is everyone who does not abide by all things written in the book of the law to perform them.'" The curse of the law is spending eternity in hell. To avoid hell and go to heaven, you must have never, ever failed to obey all of the things written in the Law. Honestly, have you ever lied, cheated on a test, stolen from someone or a store, cursed, lusted in your heart, been unkind or unforgiving, gossiped, gotten drunk or had sex outside of marriage? If you have ever sinned in any of these ways, forget about Plan A—it's too late.

The Bible says "For whoever keeps the whole law and yet stumbles in one point, he has become guilty of all" (James 2:10). In other words, one strike and you're out. To illustrate, some of us may be able to leap across a narrow ravine, but getting to heaven by our deeds is like leaping across the Grand Canyon of total perfection. We all fall short. "All have sinned and fallen short of the glory of God" (Romans 3:23).

So are you ready for Plan B?

Plan B: Believe in Christ

Fortunately, God has made a way for us to go to heaven apart from our performance. It is the way of faith—believing in Jesus Christ alone. As God says in Romans 4:5, "To the one who does not work, but believes in Him (Jesus) who justifies the ungodly, his faith is credited as righteousness."

So why does God present Jesus Christ as the object of faith? Romans 5:8–9 explains, "God demonstrates His own love toward us, in that while we were yet sinners, Christ died for us. Much more then, having now been justified by His blood, we shall be saved from the wrath of God through Him." It is simple, Christ died in our place so we might be forgiven. Romans 6:23 captures our options well: "For the wages of sin is death, but the free gift of God is eternal life in Christ Jesus our Lord." Did you notice that eternal life (going to heaven) is called a "free gift"? Is there a catch? No, Jesus Himself said in John 3:16, "For God so loved the world, that He gave His only begotten Son, that whoever believes in Him shall not perish [or go to hell], but have eternal life [go to heaven]."

So how do you receive this free gift?

Receive

The Bible has some very good news regarding how to receive this free gift of eternal life. In John 1:12 we read, "But as many as received Him, to them He gave the right to become children of God, even to those who believe in His name." Receiving Christ means believing in Him as God's only Savior from your sin. He took upon Himself the penalty of your sin, which is death—that is why He had to die on the cross. But you must personally receive His work on the cross for you to have your sins forgiven and allow your entry into heaven. So just talk to God—He hears you. Admit you are not good enough and that you have sinned against Him. Then receive His solution to your sin problem. Do yourself a huge favor and don't delay this decision to receive Jesus Christ even one minute!

After you receive Christ, turn your whole life over to Him. He said that He came to give abundant life—a full and satisfying life—so you can trust Him with everything. Then get committed to a good Bible teaching church so that you can grow in your new faith.

If you have received Christ after reading this simple presentation, please let us know. We want to encourage you and send you some free information on following Jesus Christ.

APPENDIX II

♡

Information on Stronghold Ministry

Stronghold Ministry was founded by Joe and Terri Fornear to provide spiritual support and comfort to cancer patients, caretakers and others in major life crisis. We reach out through personal contact, through the internet and via telephone. Please don't hesitate to call us or to refer someone who wants or needs some spiritual help! We want to be in your corner!

Services

We provide counseling; host support groups; speak in home groups, Sunday school classes and youth groups and Joe can be a guest speaker at your church service. We host retreats and conferences as well.

We offer our services free to cancer patients and those in crisis. Stronghold Ministry operates solely on donations. We have incorporated as a nonprofit in the State of Texas and have been granted 501(c) 3 tax exemption status by the IRS, so donations are tax deductible. Stronghold Ministry has chosen to join ECFA, The Evangelical Council for Financial Accountability, which oversees the financial practices of nonprofit organizations.

APPENDIX III

♡

Contact Information

Website
www.mystronghold.org

E-mail
jfor@mystronghold.org

Phone
214-221-7007

Joe and Terri Fornear blog
www.mystronghold.org/Blog/

Mailing address
Stronghold Ministry
P.O. Box 38478
Dallas, TX 75238